OXFORD

UNIVERSITY PRESS

KT-528-303

Great Clarendon Street, Oxford OX2 6DP

Oxford University Press is a department of the University of Oxford.
It furthers the University's objective of excellence in research, scholarship,
and education by publishing worldwide in

Oxford New York

Auckland Cape Town Dar es Salaam Hong Kong Karachi
Kuala Lumpur Madrid Melbourne Mexico City Nairobi
New Delhi Shanghai Taipei Toronto

With offices in

Argentina Austria Brazil Chile Czech Republic France Greece
Guatemala Hungary Italy Japan Poland Portugal Singapore
South Korea Switzerland Thailand Turkey Ukraine Vietnam

Oxford is a registered trade mark of Oxford University Press
in the UK and in certain other countries

Published in the United States
by Oxford University Press Inc., New York

© Oxford University Press, 2008

The moral rights of the author have been asserted
Database right Oxford University Press (maker)

First published 2008

British Library Cataloguing in Publication Data

Data available

Library of Congress Cataloguing in Publication Data

Data available

ISBN 978-0-19-921138-8 (Pbk.)

10 9 8 7 6 5 4 3 2

Typeset in Plantin
by Cepha Imaging Pvt. Ltd., Bangalore, India
Printed in China
on acid-free paper by
Asia Pacific Offset

While every effort has been made to ensure that the contents of this book are as complete,
accurate and up-to-date as possible at the date of writing, Oxford University Press is not able
to give any guarantee or assurance that such is the case. Readers are urged to take appropriately
qualified medical advice in all cases. The information in this book is intended to be useful to
the general reader, but should not be used as a means of self-diagnosis or for the prescription of
medication. The authors and the publishers do not accept responsibility or legal liability for any
errors in the text or for the misuse or misapplication of material in this book.

the**facts**

Osteoarthritis

ELIZABETH ARDEN
Chronic Pain Specialist Nurse
Hampshire Primary Care Trust, UK

DR NIGEL ARDEN
Professor and consultant Rheumatologist
Biomedical Research unit
University of Oxford and MRC Epidemiology Research Centre
Southampton University Hospitals NHS Trust
Southampton UK.

DR DAVID HUNTER
Chief of Research, New England Baptist Hospital, and
Assistant Professor of Medicine
Boston University School of Medicine
Boston, USA

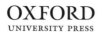

OXFORD
UNIVERSITY PRESS

Published and forthcoming titles in
thefacts series

2/
1 c

1?

the**facts**

Osteoarthritis

*To all those whose lives are affected by osteoarthritis and to our friends
and family, especially 'Joseph Badger, Dick, and Babs'
and our lovely 'Emily and Lottie'*

NA, EA

*To all the patients that I have had the opportunity to care for,
thank you for the privilege.*

*To David's adoring and beautiful wife Jo and four fantastic children
(Jordan, Sam, Charlie, and Hannah)
thank you for giving me a full and complete life,
and for understanding when my obsession with my profession
compromises our time together.*

*To my friends, colleagues, and family who read and edited this book,
thank you for your help and encouragement.*

DH

Contents

Introduction

Osteoarthritis is an increasingly common problem in our community. Many individuals with arthritis are affected by pain, stiffness or some loss of function, and are dealing with a disease that is long-lasting. We (the authors) strongly believe that the crux of any successful treatment is empowering patients with the knowledge and skills they need to help themselves. This kind of self-management approach to treating osteoarthritis is what we want to encourage the readers of this book to take up. It means actively taking charge of your own health by knowing as much as you can about osteoarthritis, and finding out how it can be best managed.

First, if you want to take charge of your own treatment, you need to understand the disease processes that can cause osteoarthritic symptoms. Part 1 details what osteoarthritis is and gives information about what causes it, who it affects, what symptoms are associated with osteoarthritis, how it is diagnosed and the long-term outlook.

Then Part 2 explains the many potential aspects of management that can be used for osteoarthritis. This includes explaining what self-management strategies are, the range of health professionals that may assist you in managing your osteoarthritis and a description of exercise, diet, all the different medicines that are used, their efficacy and their side-effects, surgical treatments and what alternative therapies there are.

Informing yourself about what conventional medical treatments are available to treat osteoarthritis is empowering. It is also important to know which healthcare practitioners (including doctors, physiotherapists, dietitians, etc.) are involved in osteoarthritis treatment so you that know who can help when particular problems arise.

There is a wealth of information on complementary treatments for arthritis. Some of these treatments are helpful, others less so. Most importantly, you should be aware of those that are likely to be of benefit and those that may do harm.

Unfortunately, many people with osteoarthritis are encouraged to rest, or they are provided with a tablet as the only means of helping their pain. However, there is a great deal of scientific research that commends the importance of exercise and a well-balanced diet in managing osteoarthritis. Personal issues such as pain management, fatigue, depression and relationships can be serious for someone with arthritis, and managing these well can make a big difference.

If you want to find out more, there's also information in the 'Useful addresses' section on what other resources are out there that may help you, such as support groups and websites.

Finally, it is important to note that this book is not intended to be a substitute for appropriate medical care. Rather, it is an opportunity for people with osteoarthritis to educate and empower themselves with tools that will help reduce their suffering.

Part 1

The background to osteoarthritis

1

What is osteoathritis?

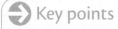 **Key points**

- Osteoarthritis is the most common type of joint disorder.

- It is a chronic condition of the synovial joint causing pain and stiffness and sometimes inflammation and swelling.

- It results in the loss of cartilage, and involves all of the structures of the joint.

- It can affect people to varying degrees, but has a large impact on the medical and financial state as it is so common.

- It is important to understand as much as possible about the condition as this will help in future management of the osteoarthritis.

Arthritis

There are over 200 different types of arthritis that can affect joints in the body, but osteoarthritis is the most common type of joint disorder in the world today, affecting the majority of those of us over the age of 65. In America it is thought this amounts to a staggering 23 million people and due to the increasing size of the elderly population and obesity in the western world this figure is likely to increase in number.

Although the disease is common, the degree to how it can affect us in our lives varies enormously between individuals. For some, osteoarthritis can have a detrimental impact on their lives while for others the condition may be little more than an inconvenience.

3

The history of osteoarthritis

Osteoarthritis is not a new disease – in fact it has been around for many years. Scientists examining the skeletons of humans and mammals from as long ago as the ice age discovered that joints had osteoarthritis.

What does osteoarthritis mean?

Like many other medical conditions, osteoarthritis has been acknowledged as a disease for hundreds of years and its name is derived from the Latin language. When the name is translated 'osteo' means bone, 'arthro' means joints and 'itis' means inflammation. Therefore 'osteoarthritis' means inflammation of the bones in the joint. In reality the bone does not become inflamed, but the joint as a whole can as a result of the disease process. It continues to be called osteoarthritis (or OA when abbreviated).

What is osteoarthritis?

Over the past years musculoskeletal scientists and clinicians have deliberated over the correct definition of osteoarthritis. They concluded that it is a chronic condition of the synovial joint that develops over time and is the result of the thinning or loss of the cartilage, which is found at the ends of the bones. This loss of cartilage causes a reduced joint space, and sometimes the bone ends come into direct contact with each other, which in turn causes pain and anatomical changes to the bone itself in addition to the other structures of the joint. For this reason osteoarthritis is now recognized as a disease of the whole joint.

Osteoarthritis – a chronic disease

A chronic condition differs from that of an acute illness, such as appendicitis or the flu, in that an acute illness has a start and an end to the illness, often with a treatment in the middle. A chronic condition often has a more gradual onset as opposed to an immediate response to trauma, it is often ongoing and may never end. Diabetes, heart disease and hypertension are also chronic conditions like osteoarthritis that develop gradually over time and continue to persist.

When the term 'disease' is used in this context it does not mean osteoarthritis is contagious or the result of injury, but that it is a recognized medical disorder that is accompanied by symptoms and clinical signs and follows a natural process.

The joints affected by osteoarthritis

The joints that are most prone to osteoarthritis tend to be the weight-bearing joints of the body: the knee, hip and back. In addition it can also commonly affect digits of the hand. Other joints such as the ankle and shoulder and elbow are less likely to develop osteoarthritis unless there has been previous trauma to that joint.

What are the signs and symptoms of osteoarthritis?

The symptoms for those who have osteoarthritis consist of pain and stiffness (the latter is often relieved in a few minutes by movement) in the affected joints, although it varies between individuals. In some cases the pain can lead to reduced movement, which in turn limits the function of the joint. In severe cases inflammation can develop causing the joint to become swollen and warm. The signs that clinicians identify as part of the osteoarthritis condition include swelling and bony enlargement around the joint and crepitus (creaking of the joint when moved).

The joint with osteoarthritis

The synovial joint is made up of two bones' ends, a layer of cartilage lining the end of each bone, a capsule lined by synovium which produces synovial fluid, ligaments, tendons and muscles (Fig. 1.1). The role of cartilage, which when healthy is usually smooth, firm, white and rubbery in nature, is to help the bone ends move smoothly and painlessly against each other when the joint is moved. The cartilage also acts as a shock absorber.

Synovial fluid is a viscous fluid of a similar consistency to car engine oil: it helps the joint ends move easily by acting as a lubricant. As a result we move joints easily, often without noticing the action.

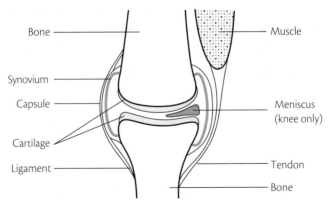

Figure 1.1 The normal synovial joint without osteoarthritis.

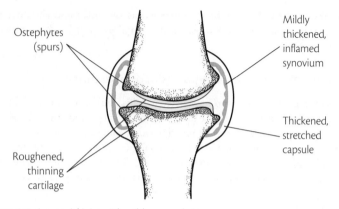

Figure 1.2 A synovial joint with mild osteoarthritis.

The tendons attach the muscles to bone and are involved in moving and stabilizing the joints. The ligaments attach the two bones together and help to stabilize the joint at rest and during movement.

The bone tissue and cartilage are always undergoing regeneration and as long as this continues the joints work smoothly together. However, if the cartilage starts to diminish in size then it can put strain on the other tissues and as a result they work overtime in trying to compensate.

The joint with mild osteoarthritis

Figure 1.2 shows a joint with mild osteoarthritic changes. As you can see, over time the cartilage has become thinner, scantier and less smooth in appearance which means that the two bones do not move as smoothly during joint movement. The space between the bone ends has also become narrower due to the thinning of the cartilage, and as a result more pressure is put on the tendons and ligaments to maintain joint stability. The bone in response to the depleted cartilage and imbalance starts to grow little bony spurs called osteophytes.

The joint with severe osteoarthritis

You can see in Figure 1.3 that there is now much greater cartilage loss, including areas where the cartilage has disappeared exposing the underlying bones. The osteophytes are now bigger, and the end of the bones starts to thicken in response to the increased stresses that it encounters due to the loss of the shock-absorbing effect of the overlying cartilage. As the cartilage breaks down debris can be found in the synovial fluid, which is struggling to produce enough lubricant for the bone ends and remaining cartilage.

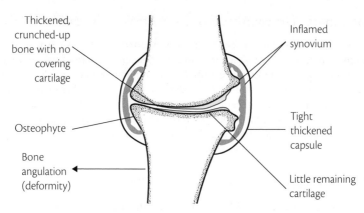

Figure 1.3 A synovial joint with severe osteoarthritis.

This advanced stage of osteoarthritis results in pain and stiffness and inflammation as the joint struggles to maintain its smooth function.

Other names for osteoarthritis

'Wear and tear', 'degenerative changes', ' osteoarthrosis', 'degenerative joint disease', 'degenerative arthritis' and 'decaying cartilage' are all common expressions used by physicians when describing osteoarthritis to a patient, however they all mean osteoarthritis. Some of these can sound quite catastrophic and are inaccurate, but unfortunately many people continue to use them even though they sound very alarming.

What about rheumatoid arthritis and osteoporosis?

Medical conditions and their names can be very confusing, and sometimes people get muddled about the difference between rheumatoid arthritis, osteoporosis and osteoarthritis. They are all rheumatological conditions, but they are very different diseases.

- *Rheumatoid arthritis* (RA) is a condition where the synovium becomes inflamed and causes severe damage to the cartilage and bone. It is less common than osteoarthritis, presents with different signs and symptoms and its treatment is quite different to osteoarthritis.

- *Osteoporosis* is a disease of bones leading to an increased risk of fracture. It does not affect the joints and rarely causes joint pain. Its treatment by physicians is quite different to that of osteoarthritis.

The impact of osteoarthritis in the general population

Osteoarthritis is common, especially in the elderly, and as such it causes strains to both the medical services and the financial welfare of the country. For example, in the USA it accounts for 315 million visits to the doctor per year, approximately 744,000 hospital admissions per year and amounts to 68 million days off work. In recent years osteoarthritis has been seen as the second biggest cause of work disability in those aged 50 and over, ischaemic heart disease being in first position, and therefore is of major concern, as it has significant implications on the welfare state.

The impact of osteoarthritis to each individual

Of course not everybody with osteoarthritis will have to visit a doctor or be admitted to hospital, and not everybody will stop work due to the condition. As you will discover in this book, osteoarthritis affects people to different levels. For some osteoarthritis can have a major impact on their lifestyle, but for many it may cause just a minor disruption and some people have virtually no symptoms at all, often unaware that they have signs of osteoarthritis. For some people the disease only affects the one joint whilst for others the disease can be widespread and continue to progress, so affecting movement, causing pain and distress and impacting on private and working lifestyles, sometimes leading to surgical treatments. We are all individuals, and our experience of osteoarthritis will vary.

In summary

Osteoarthritis is a chronic or long-term disease of the synovial joints characterized by a loss or depletion of cartilage and associated with pain and stiffness. The impact and experiences of osteoarthritis varies between individuals: however, the one thing clinicians know is that the more information people have about their osteoarthritis the easier it is to manage.

2

Why do we get osteoarthritis?

Key points

- Research plays a key role in helping us understand why we get osteoarthritis.

- There are some general factors affecting our joints and also some specific factors that increase our risk of developing osteoarthritis.

- Some factors we have no control over (age, genetics) but others, such as fitness and obesity, we are able to modulate.

- The more we understand the reasons why we develop osteoarthritis, the easier it is to accept the condition and manage it.

We now know from the previous chapter that osteoarthritis (OA) is a chronic condition, characterized by well-defined changes on X-ray and associated with pain and joint stiffness: but why do we develop it? Clinicians and research scientists have, over the past couple of decades, studied people who have been diagnosed with osteoarthritis. The research has focused on the following areas:

- Lifestyles, which include the nature of current or previous type of work, type of diet, and level of activity throughout life.

- Past medical histories including injuries to joints, previous surgery and other medical conditions.

- Family history, examining osteoarthritis within families to establish if there are any connections to it having a genetic connection.

By studying these three main areas researchers have gained insight into the factors that can influence the development of osteoarthritis in individuals.

These influential factors are called risk factors in the medical profession and they can be split into two main groups:

1. 'Systemic' or general risk factors that can affect any joint developing OA. These include age, genetics, bone density, nutrition and ethnic group.

2. 'Local' risk factors that affect specific joints of the body such as obesity, trauma and congenital medical conditions.

Although several risk factors have been identified for osteoarthritis, like many other chronic conditions there is not always one single factor that is responsible for the disease – for example, you could be overweight and also have a family history of osteoarthritis. Coronary heart disease is a good example of this as it too has many risk factors associated with its onset: smoking, diabetes, stress, obesity, high cholesterol levels, lack of fitness, genetic make-up and so on. Patients presenting with coronary heart disease are often found to have more than one of these risk factors.

The aim of this chapter is to examine the risk factors that can influence the disease onset and progression of osteoarthritis, and in so doing hopefully answer some of your questions and address some of the myths surrounding the cause of osteoarthritis.

Systemic risk factors – general factors affecting any joint

These risk factors tend to define the ability of the joints to stay healthy and repair themselves in response to injury or repetitive trauma such as sports or occupation. A person with no systemic risk factors can work in high-risk occupations or participate in high-risk sports, such as professional football, without developing OA, whereas a person with several risk factors may develop OA in low-risk occupations or without participating in any high-risk sports.

Age

Probably the most obvious finding and well-known observation of osteoarthritis is that it is generally uncommon in young people and becomes very common as we all get older. It is thought that by the time we reach the age of 75 years there is a 90 per cent chance of having osteoarthritis on X-ray somewhere in the body. There are two main reasons why age is such a strong risk factor:

1. *Inability of the body to repair cartilage.* During our lives the joints are working constantly, which is healthy and quite normal, but it does mean that they have

been under a large cumulative joint strain over the years. The cartilage, which acts as the shock absorber, diminishes in size (osteoarthritis) and becomes unable to repair itself. It is thought this inability of the body to repair the cartilage is due to the reduction of growth hormones. Growth hormones are necessary for cartilage turnover but as we age they are reduced as part of the ageing process and the body loses its ability to repair the cartilage.

2. *Changes to our activity and fitness levels.* It is recognized that as we get older our general fitness decreases, which in turn affects the muscle strength. Muscles are needed to support the joints both above and below a joint: however, when the muscle strength is diminished or reduced, then greater pressure is placed on the joint itself, in particular the cartilage.

Although the prevalence of osteoarthritis increases sharply with age there are still some people who do not develop it. Scientists believe this may occur because there are protective mechanisms in place and/or that there are no other risk factors to influence its onset.

Genetics

The latest evidence to date indicates that half of the risk of developing osteoarthritis of the hand, hip and knee can be attributed to genetic factors. This was first realized for hand OA when doctors noticed that most patients had a family member with the same condition. It is very unlikely that there is a single gene that determines the genetic risk, but rather a large number of genes. The genes that have been examined are those responsible for the make-up of cartilage and bone, however it is likely that genes determining joint shape, muscle strength and body weight will also have important roles to play. However, as previously mentioned, there are other important risk factors for developing osteoarthritis and these may modify our genetic risk of developing OA.

Gender

Until the age of 55 years osteoarthritis affects men and women equally; however, after the age of 55 women are twice as likely to develop osteoarthritis, particularly at the hand and knee. As most women are postmenopausal after the age of 55, it is suggested the drop of oestrogen levels is the factor responsible for its higher prevalence in women above this age. Research has shown hormone replacement therapy can slow or delay the onset of osteoarthritis, but unfortunately it does not prevent the progression of the condition. As hormone replacement therapy is associated with other medical health risks if taken for prolonged periods (heart attack and thrombosis and increased risk of breast cancer) it is not routinely seen as a treatment choice for osteoarthritis.

Bone density

Research has shown that there is a link between bone density and osteoarthritis. Those people who have a high bone density are more at risk of osteoarthritis whilst those with a low bone density are less at risk. Therefore if you have osteoporosis you are less likely to develop osteoarthritis. It is thought this could be because the bones are lighter and more compliant in osteoporosis and therefore put less strain on the cartilage leading to less wear and tear. This is not to say that osteoporosis is a good disease to develop, as it has serious health risks associated with it.

Ethnic groups

Generally speaking osteoarthritis is prevalent in all ethnic groups around the world. However, American research has shown the rates of osteoarthritis are generally lower in places where obesity is lower such as China and Asia. There hip osteoarthritis and hand osteoarthritis are found to be one-tenth and one-half of the numbers found in white Americans, respectively. As the prevalence is lower in these parts of the world it is thought that there may also be some genetic or other systemic factor that protects them from the development of this condition.

Studies comparing the rates of osteoarthritis between black and white Americans in the hip and knee joint found that although the rates were similar, knee involvement was more common in black Americans, probably due to a higher body mass index.

Nutrition

It has generally been thought that vitamins have played a role in the health of our joints for many decades and there is now evidence to suggest that they do have a beneficial role to play, especially in the knee joint. It is suggested that a diet lacking in either vitamin C, D or E can affect the health of the joint and cause osteoarthritis. When the cartilage is broken down in osteoarthritis, free oxygen radicals (produced by chondrocytes in damaged cartilage) are released. These cause oxidative damage to the cartilage that is left and also the other joint tissue so leading to progression of osteoarthritis. Vitamins C and E are antioxidants (the antidotes) and therefore have a beneficial role in collagen synthesis and joint health. In fact one study found those with a diet rich in vitamin C had less knee pain and slower progression of osteoarthritis.

Vitamin D has an important role in bone metabolism and may improve the metabolism of the periarticular bone (bone ends) in response to excess loading and joint damage. It may also have direct beneficial effects on cartilage and improve muscle function and hence stabilize the joint more effectively. Studies of people who have high serum levels of vitamin D or high dietary intake of vitamin D have demonstrated a protective effect in subjects with knee osteoarthritis.

Local mechanical risk factors – factors that influence the onset in specific joints

Injury

It has now been shown that previous injuries to joints can be a risk factor for developing osteoarthritis in later years. Acute injuries such as meniscal (cartilage) and anterior cruciate (ligaments in the knee) tears and dislocations increase the risk of osteoarthritis in later years in the joint in question. In general a severe injury of any joint may be followed by osteoarthritis in later years but you are more susceptible if you already have osteoarthritis of another joint.

Athletes such as footballers and rugby players are prone to such injuries and often go on to develop osteoarthritis in later years in those joints where the injury took place. Unfortunately, although surgery can correct injuries at the time it does not completely reduce the risks of developing osteoarthritis in the operated joint. It is reassuring to know that today in school and at fitness clubs great emphasis is made on stretching and warming up and cooling down so as to reduce the likehood of such injuries.

Repetitive strain on joints – wear and tear

Generally speaking moderate exercise is extremely good for your physical and mental health and does not cause osteoarthritis in later years. As parents we are often telling our children 'everything in moderation is good for you'. There is no evidence that recreational running or sports lead to an increased risk of OA. However, there are groups of people such as athletes who train at very high and intense levels causing extra stress to joints and exposing themselves to injury and in so doing increasing their risk of osteoarthritis in later years. This is mainly true of professional weightlifters, footballers and rugby players.

There are also groups of people in whom evidence shows that repeated joint loading with some activities can increase the risk of osteoarthritis in later years. For instance osteoarthritis of the knee is more common in the Chinese female population who squat excessively as part of their culture (this despite a low body weight), osteoarthritis is more common in the hands of cotton mill workers who put extra stress on their finger joints, and osteoarthritis of the hip joint is common amongst farmers (due to a combination of lifting heavy loads and walking on uneven ground).

Muscle strength and weakness

Generally speaking good muscle strength is vital for a healthy joint, and some joints have even been shown to have a lower rate of osteoarthritis when supported well. For example, strong quadriceps has been shown to reduce the risk of knee osteoarthritis. However, there are some areas of the body that can increase the risk of osteoarthritis if the muscle strength is good. Bus drivers, for example, are prone to osteoarthritis as they have a very tight hand grip.

Joint deformity

There are some congenital abnormalities that can increase the risk of osteoarthritis in later years. These are usually conditions of the musculo-skeletal system where excess stress is placed on joints due to abnormalities of the joint tissues or bones, which results in dysfunctional joints. Examples of this are acetabular dysplasia, and slipped capital femoral epiphysis which are characterized by abnormal shapes of the hip joint.

Obesity

Being overweight is a major concern for health professionals managing all chronic diseases, heart disease and diabetes to name but two. Not surprisingly, being overweight causes extra stress on the weight-bearing joints such as the hip and knee and results in an accelerated rate of osteoarthritis. It is suggested that for every extra pound of body weight your knees carry an alarming three pounds of extra stress!! The effects of being overweight have a direct effect on the stress of the joint but are also linked to metabolic changes that can affect the risk of developing hand osteoarthritis. Studies have shown obesity to be the biggest risk factor for developing osteoarthritis of the knee, but weight loss can reduce the risk of subsequent knee osteoarthritis.

Conclusion

There are many risk factors associated with osteoarthritis and the more risk factors that you have, the higher the chance you will develop osteoarthritis. However, just because you have one risk factor it does not automatically lead you to develop osteoarthritis.

There are some risk factors that we are at present unable to alter, for instance ageing and our genetic make-up. However, there are some risk factors that we can influence, for instance we can alter our lifestyles to encourage a healthy weight and maintain an optimal level of exercise in order to reduce our chances of developing osteoarthritis.

Research is always continuing into this field of osteoarthritis, and it is hoped that with a better understanding of the different risk factors responsible for the onset of the disease in years to come clinicians will be able to develop some breakthroughs and practice preventative medicine. As individuals it is hoped we will be able to play an active role in minimizing the onset of osteoarthritis.

3

Joints and osteoarthritis

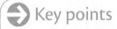 Key points

- Osteoarthritis affects the synovial joints, such as the knee, hip and fingers.

- The joint contains many structures including bone, cartilage, muscles, synovium, ligaments and tendons.

- Osteoarthritis can affect all of these structures and is therefore a condition of the whole joint.

Joints are part of the body's musculo-skeletal system which consists of 212 bones and soft tissue that accounts for over half our body mass. It is a vast system consisting of bones, muscles, tendons, ligaments, cartilage, synovial fluid, blood vessels and nerves, all of which work together to provide a system vital for our daily physical needs.

In order to understand the process of osteoarthritis it is helpful to have some knowledge of this complex system and how it works. It is easier to follow your management plan if you have a good understanding of some of the mechanisms behind osteoarthritis.

Types of joints

We have over 200 joints in our body. They vary in their structural make-up and in their movement range, but essentially a joint is where two bone ends come together. Structurally some are more complex than others and for this reason they have been categorized into three groups:

1. Fibrous (e.g. the skull).

2. Cartilaginous.(e.g. the rib cage).

3. Synovial (e.g. the knee or the hip).

We tend to think that all joints move but although most joints do, there are some joints that have no movement or only a little movement. For this reason they are categorized into one of the following groups:

1. Synarthroses (not able to move).

2. Ampiarthrosis (slight movement).

3. Diarthroses (freely moveable).

Synovial joints are affected by osteoarthritis and they are nearly always the diarthrosis type of joint. This chapter will now look at this type of joint in more detail.

The normal synovial joint

Most joints of the body are synovial joints and due to their structure are the most freely moveable joints in the skeletal system. The movements of these joints vary according to the different shapes of the bones and subsequently fall into one of the groups as listed below and as shown in Figure 3.1:

(a) plane joints (mid-tarsal – the joints in the arch of the foot)

(b) hinge joints (the elbow and ankle)

(c) condyloid joint (the knuckles and wrist joints)

(d) ball and socket (the shoulder and hip)

(e) pivot joint (top of the lower arm)

(f) saddle joint (the base of the thumb).

Despite having varying movements synovial joints all share the same structural make-up. Each joint has bone, cartilage, ligaments, synovial fluid, muscles, a capsule and a blood and nerve supply. These structures work together to enable a joint to move smoothly and freely.

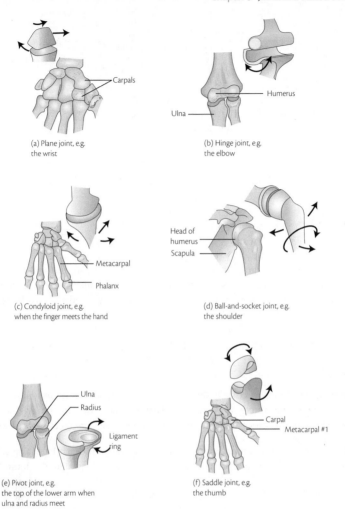

Figure 3.1 The classification of synovial joints. (a) the plane joint; (b) the hinge joint; (c) the condyloid joint; (d) the ball and socket joint; (e) the pivot joint; (f) the saddle joint.

The mechanism of a typical synovial joint

In a synovial joint the ends of the bones are covered by cartilage, which prevents the bones from rubbing against each other and also acts as a cushion and shock absorber. When the joint is moving synovial fluid bathes the cartilage and helps the structures to glide over each other without causing any friction.

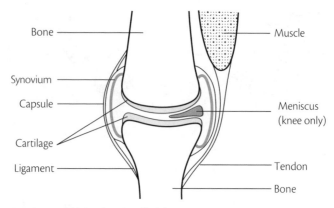

Figure 3.2 A synovial joint showing all of the structures.

The muscles and ligaments work hard to keep the joint in line and prevent it from dislocating and the sensory nerves relay messages regarding pain or stretching back to the brain. These structures of the synovial joint work together, each having a unique role to play.

Structures of the synovial joint

Cartilage

Cartilage is whitish in colour, strong, dense and rubbery in nature, and serves several important functions. As well as playing a role within the synovial joint it gives shape to our noses and ears and also supports the airways and vocal cords.

The type of cartilage found in the synovial joint is hyaline cartilage, also called articular cartilage (hence some clinicians call these joints articular joints). In the synovial joint its major role is to act as a shock absorber, cushioning the gaps between the bone ends, and also allowing joint surfaces to glide freely over each other. It is made up of a lattice framework of collagens (structural proteins), which contains proteoglycans (proteins attached to complex carbohydrates and amino acids) and water. Within the cartilage are chondrocytes, the cells that are responsible for the synthesis of new cartilage and also the maintenance of the quality of the existing cartilage. In our lives there are constant changes taking place with the structure of our cartilage and these chondrocytes are responsible for keeping things in equilibrium.

In OA the chondrocytes are unable to keep pace with the breakdown of cartilage and hence it becomes scanty and depleted. Unfortunately the cartilage does not have its own blood supply and so relies on the synovial fluid to bathe it with nutrients and rid it of toxins and waste products. This process takes place when the joint is moving.

The knee contains two menisci, which are pieces of fibro-cartilage that act as spacers and shock absorbers to help the two ends of the bones to maintain a large contact surface area and spread the load. They are often torn in sports injuries and referred to as a 'torn cartilage'.

Synovial fluid

This is the fluid found within the joint: its appearance is similar to raw egg white. It originates form the synovial membrane and it is the product of filtered blood, but it also contains special glycoproteins (proteins and carbohydrates attached) that give it the slippery characteristics it needs. The fluid sits in the joint cavity but when the joint is under pressure the movements force the fluid in and out of the hyaline cartilage: this helps keep the cartilage healthy as it delivers nutrients and disposes of waste products with this action.

The joint cavity

This is the space within the joint that holds a small amount of synovial fluid.

The articular capsule

This is the name given to two layers of connective tissue that surround the structures of the joint. The outer layer is continuous with the bone and the inner layer is called the synovial membrane. The aim of the capsule is to keep every structure contained within the joint together.

Ligaments

Synovial joints are reinforced with ligaments that help stabilize the structure as a whole and prevent dislocation by preventing excessive or unwanted movements. Generally the more ligaments a joint has the more secure and stronger it becomes. Ligaments are limited in that they can only stretch up to 6 per cent of their normal length.

Nerves and blood vessels

The synovial joint as a whole is supplied with both sensory nerves and blood vessels. The role of the sensory nerves is to both sense pain and to sense how much stretching is taking place within the joint. Without these sensory nerves we would move the joints in unsafe directions and cause injury, thus they have a protective role to play. The blood vessels are found in the synovial membrane and provide nutrients to the synovium and capsule in addition to producing the synovial fluid for the joint.

Muscles and tendons

Muscles play an important role in the musculo-skeletal system as they help maintain posture, produce movement and also generate heat. There are many in the body and they come in varying shapes and sizes. Muscles consist of muscle tissue and connective tissue and they all have a nerve and blood supply.

The tendons are rope-like pieces of strong fibrous tissue that join the muscles to the bones. They play a very important role in moving the joint in its intended direction, and also in stabilizing the joint during activities such as standing. For a tendon to work well it needs good muscle tone which will keep the tendon taught (even when the muscle is not under stress): without this the tendon would be loose and the joint could move in directions not intended for it and produce injury.

Bones

The bones of our skeleton come in varying shapes and sizes, which enable them to carry out important functions such as support (the legs support the upper body), protection (the skull), store of minerals (calcium and phosphate) and blood cell formation. In the moving (diarthroses) synovial joint they act as levers.

Bones have a rich blood supply and are very active metabolically with up to 10 per cent of our skeleton being remodelled every year. Anatomically they are closely related to the hyaline cartilage because it sits directly on the ends of the bone. Scientists studying OA have observed a close relationship between the bone and cartilage: as one changes its structure so the other one responds in order to compensate.

The synovial joint with osteoarthritis

The most prominent feature of any synovial joint with osteoarthritis is the fraying and loss of cartilage. The fraying of the superficial cartilage reduces the ability of the bone ends to glide over each other, which often results in the bone feeling stiffer and occasionally sticking during movement. The loss of cartilage reduces the distance between the bone ends which means the ligaments are often less taut so that the joint often feels unstable. Other physiological changes take place in a natural attempt to correct the depletion of cartilage or in direct response to the loss.

As the cartilage becomes depleted the bone beneath it becomes thicker and denser. In an attempt to compensate for the loss of cartilage the bone starts to grow new bone called osteophytes. These develop around the edge of the damaged or depleted cartilage region and are spur-shaped. In advanced OA with total loss of cartilage, bone cysts can develop. It is thought this happens because there is no longer a buffer to stop the synovial fluid entering and leaving the bone: this fluid then reacts with the bone marrow and cysts are formed.

The synovium also changes its appearance in OA and can become thicker, bulkier and occasionally inflamed. This may be caused in part by cartilage debris that has accumulated in the joint as it is shed from the articular surface. The thickened, inflamed synovium produces more synovial fluid than normal, which accumulates in the joint leading to swelling of the joint.

As a result of pain, the muscles around the joint tend to waste and become weaker. This, when combined with the reduced tautness of the ligaments, often increases instability of the joint. As is evident from the above description, OA of the joint does not just affect the cartilage but affects all the different structures of the joint.

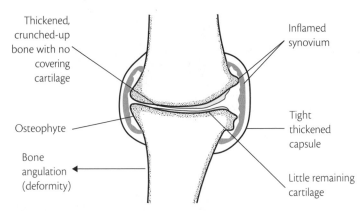

Figure 3.3 A synovial joint with severe osteoarthritis.

Common sites of osteoarthritis

Although in theory osteoarthritis can affect any synovial joint in the body, the most commonly affected joints are the knees, hips and hands and less commonly the shoulder, spine, ankles and feet.

Knee osteoarthritis

This weight-bearing joint is the most complex and the largest joint of the body, and has many structures in place to keep it stable.

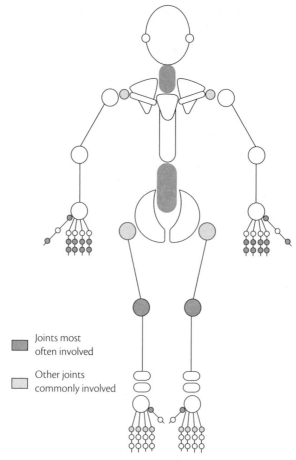

Figure 3.4 The joints affected by osteoarthritis.

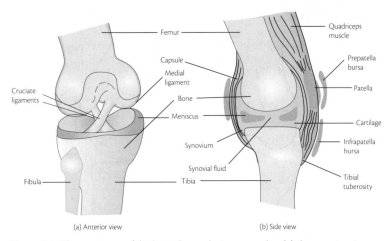

Figure 3.5 The structures of the knee that make it so complex: (a) the anterior view (front); (b) the side view.

It consists of three major sections (Figure 3.6), all of which can be affected by OA. The progression of OA in this joint is usually slow, often taking several years and frequently not appearing until in the fifth decade of life, unless a previous knee injury has taken place. The good news is that the condition can remain stable for many years without worsening of symptoms.

Hip osteoarthritis

The hip, as a 'ball and socket' joint, has a wide range of movement and also carries a great deal of the body's weight, making it prone to OA. The pattern as to its development varies enormously between individuals, but it is thought that a period of between three months and three years of symptoms precedes advanced OA that necessitates surgery. There are three areas of this joint that can be affected by osteoarthritis.

Hand osteoarthritis

Osteoarthritis of the hand usually affects the distal interphalangeal (DIP) (the farthest joint of the finger) and the proximal interphalangeal (PIP) (the middle joint of the finger) joint and also the thumb base joint (Figure 3.7).

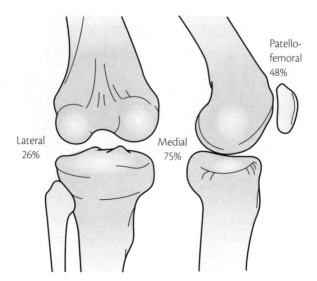

Figure 3.6 The knee joint showing the areas most commonly affected by osteoarthritis.

In the fingers, it usually starts with an ache in the affected joint which tends to come and go in the initial years. This is then followed by warm and tender joints during which time the bone ends can become enlarged. After several years of this the swellings become firm and fixed and the joint can lose some of its movement. These are often referred to as Heberden's nodes on the DIP joint and Bouchard's nodes on the PIP joint (Figure 3.8). Once mature they are often relatively painless. Following this it is often common for the OA to progress no further.

The spine

The spine consists of 33 vertebrae: 7 cervical, 12 thoracic, 5 lumbar and 5 sacral. Each vertebra can vary in size but they are all connected by ligaments, tendons, muscles and discs. The vertebra are not synovial joints and therefore officially do not develop OA.

Facet joints of the spine can develop OA as they are synovial joints. If we feel down the back of our spines we will feel the facet joints. They are the joints that enable the vertebrae to stack one on top of the other. Over time the hyaline cartilage can fray and deplete resulting in osteophytes. In theory it could happen to any of the facet joints, but the most likely to be affected by OA are

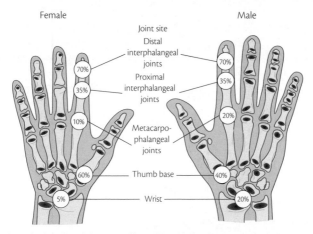

Figure 3.7 The hand and the sites affected by osteoarthritis in men and in women.

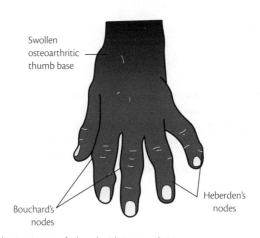

Figure 3.8 A classic picture of a hand with osteoarthritis.

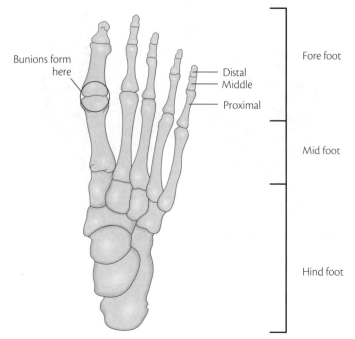

Bunions form here

Distal
Middle
Proximal

Fore foot

Mid foot

Hind foot

Figure 3.9 The skeletal structure of the foot.

the cervical and the lumbar facet (the areas of the spine that allow movement and enable us to bend and lean back). In advanced OA of the facets the loss of cushioning from the cartilage and the loss of disc height (a common feature of ageing) can cause pressure on the nerves, which can then cause nerve pain (sharp, burning, stabbing) or numbness and pins and needles. In severe cases this results in spinal stenosis in which the nerves are severely compromised.

Shoulder

This is a freely moving ball and socket joint and consists of the humerus (upper arm), clavicle (collar bone) and scapular bones (shoulder blade). Large muscles from the back help support the joint and aid the upper arm movements. OA of the shoulder is uncommon and it often develops as a result of previous trauma, chronic inflammation or excessive over use, for example in sportsmen and women.

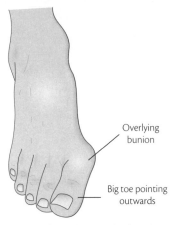

Overlying
bunion

Big toe pointing
outwards

Figure 3.10 A foot with osteoarthritis showing the formation of a bunion.

Feet

Our feet work hard through out our lives supporting most of our body weight. Considering the risk factors for developing OA, it is not surprisingly that it is present in 50 per cent of those aged 75 and over. The foot is made up of 26 bones and is divided into three areas: the hindfoot (ankle), the midfoot (the tarsal bones) and the forefoot (toes) (Figure 3.9).

OA of the foot commonly affects the first metatarsal (great toe joint) joint, the subtalar (between ankle and heel bone) joint and the ankle joint. Bunions and hammer toes commonly develop as a result of OA (Figure 3.10).

The elbow

This is a hinge joint that just allows two types of movement: extension (moving away from the body) and flexion (moving towards the body). It is uncommon to get OA in this joint unless it has been subjected to trauma or repeated stress, such as weight-lifting.

Conclusion

There are many different structures that make up the synovial joint and they all have a different role to play in facilitating the function of the joint. When the cartilage is depleted by OA it impacts on all the structures as they try to compensate and therefore the joint as a whole is affected.

4

What are the symptoms and signs associated with osteoarthritis?

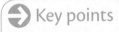 Key points

- The main symptoms associated with osteoarthritis are stiff and painful joints which impact on your ability to function.

- The main signs relate to an altered range of motion, crepitus and tenderness of the joint.

- Please seek help from a health professional to make the correct diagnosis.

Patient's perspective

EA, 57-year-old registered nurse

For me, osteoarthritis presents many challenges. The majority of those challenges are associated with the [type and amount of] pain that I experience. The osteoarthritis is most severe in my knees.

Due to this condition, I struggle with climbing stairs, coordination, standing for longer than a few minutes, standing from a sitting position. When the osteoarthritis in my knee becomes inflamed, I have trouble doing simple tasks such as bending my knee, exercising and walking normally.

Attempts have been made to ease the symptoms of my osteoarthritis. Over the course of several trips to my orthopedics office, I have received two types

of injections; those injections offered varying degrees of relief. The first
type of injection was cortisone. The dosage was administered in one shot and I
have received multiple dosages over the past several years. It only offered temporary relief, though 'temporary relief' can vary anywhere between several
hours and several days. The other injection that I received was entitled Synvisc.
Unlike the previous treatments, Synvisc didn't offer any relief for me.

Osteoarthritis is a joint disease. Unlike many other forms of arthritis that are
systemic illnesses, such as rheumatoid arthritis, scleroderma and lupus, osteoarthritis does not affect other organs of the body.

Symptoms of osteoarthritis vary greatly from person to person. Some people can be debilitated by their symptoms whereas others may have remark-
ably few symptoms in spite of the dramatic degeneration of their joints shown
on X-rays. Symptoms also can be intermittent. It is not unusual for patients
with osteoarthritis of the hands and knees to have years of pain-free intervals
between symptomatic epsiodes.

The severity of symptoms in osteoarthritis is greatly influenced by a person's
attitudes, anxiety, depression or daily activities.

The symptoms and signs of osteoarthritis will also vary depending on the joint
affected. The main symptoms associated with OA are stiff and painful joints
which impacts on your day to day function. The main signs relate to an altered
range of motion, crepitus and tenderness of the joint. This chapter explains
each of these symptoms and signs in more detail.

Please remember that the presence of one or even all of these symptoms
and signs does not mean that you have osteoarthritis – many of them can be
produced by other disorders. Please seek help from a health professional to
make the correct diagnosis and do not use this chapter for making your own
diagnosis.

The main symptoms and signs associated with osteoarthritis include pain,
stiffness, reduction of the range of movement within the joint, tenderness,
crepitus, swelling and muscle weakness.

Pain

The pain of osteoarthritis almost always begins gradually, progressing slowly
over many years. Once established, pain may behave like a roller-coaster, with
bad spells followed by periods of relative relief.

Pain usually comes from deep within the joint. It is generally described as aching, sharp or a burning pain. It is also often described as mechanical; that is, it is worse with activity such as when there is weight or resistance put on the joint/s affected (for example, walking or climbing stairs and therefore putting pressure on the knee joint). The pain is usually relieved after resting for a few minutes.

Sometimes the activity-related pain will persist after long periods of activity (playing sports, hiking, shovelling snow, working in the garden or other repeated activities of daily living) and towards the end of the day. Some people with OA say that cold and solids or humid weather may increase their pain.

As the disease advances and the structure of the joint is badly damaged, the pain may occur even when the joint is at rest, and it can keep a sufferer awake at night.

The pain of osteoarthritis usually occurs in the area of the affected joint; however, in some cases, the pain may be referred to other areas. For example, the pain of osteoarthritis of the hip may actually be felt in the knee.

Stiffness

The joint stiffness associated with osteoarthritis usually follows periods of inactivity. Usually it is at its worst in the morning on first rising from bed – lasting less than 30 minutes – and can also be troublesome after resting during the day. Moving the joint or doing some exercise for a few minutes can help shake off the stiffness associated with osteoarthritis. Usually the stiffness lasts for 2–3 minutes and is described as 'gelling'.

Reduction in the normal range of motion within the joint

As the condition causes more symptoms, the joint may become less movable and eventually it may not be possible to fully straighten or bend it.

Tenderness

Joints affected by osteoarthritis may be tender to the touch, even in the absence of obvious signs of inflammation.

Crepitus

The crunching, creaking, crackling, grating or grinding sounds and sensation on movement of the joint is called 'crepitus'. This sensation with joint movement probably occurs because osteoarthritis leads to a roughening of the normally smooth cartilage surfaces inside the joint.

Swelling

Later in the course of OA, swelling of the joint may develop. This can either be soft in consistency (due to extra synovial fluid) or firm (due to bony enlargement at the joint – most commonly seen in the joints of the fingers).

The soft joint swelling from fluid is called an effusion. An effusion results from the accumulation of excess fluid in the joint space. Potentially this swelling will be warm, but if the joint is red or hot this is unusual for osteoarthritis and you should have this checked by your doctor as it is more suggestive of other conditions such as gout, pseudogout or an infection.

Bony growths called osteophytes or bone spurs (called Heberden's or Bouchard's nodes) commonly develop in the joints at the ends or middle of the fingers. These bony protuberances can be felt under the skin near joints, and typically enlarge over time.

Muscle weakness

In more advanced osteoarthritis, muscles may become weaker because of insufficient use. In some joints (such as the knee), the ligaments, which surround and support the joint, stretch so that the joint becomes unstable.

Symptoms in specific joints

Osteoarthritis does not affect all joints equally. The condition most commonly affects the hand, knee, hip and spine, and only rarely affects the elbow, wrist and ankle (Fig 4.1).

Furthermore, osteoarthritis often has an asymmetric pattern, affecting joints on either side of the body to a different extent.

Knees

Osteoarthritis is particularly debilitating in the weight-bearing joints of the knees. Osteoarthritis of the knees is often associated with obesity or a history of repeated injury and/or joint surgery. Advanced osteoarthritis of the knee may be associated with changes in the alignment of the knee, including a bow-legged or a knock-kneed appearance. Osteoarthritis of the knee may also cause a Baker's cyst, a collection of joint fluid in the hollow at the back of the knee.

Patients with osteoarthritis of the weight-bearing joints (like the knees) sometimes develop a limp, which can worsen as the joint degenerates. Although

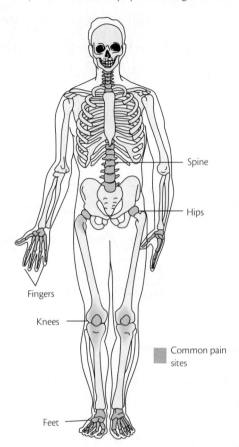

Figure 4.1 Common sites of pain in osteoarthritis.

painful, the arthritic knee usually retains reasonable flexibility. The pain of knee osteoarthritis is often made worse during activities such as walking, squatting, getting in or out of a chair and climbing stairs.

Spine

Osteoarthritis may affect the cartilage in the discs that form cushions between the bones of the spine (otherwise known as degenerative disc disease), the moving joints of the spine itself or both. Osteoarthritis typically affects the most flexible regions of the spine, including the vertebrae (the individual

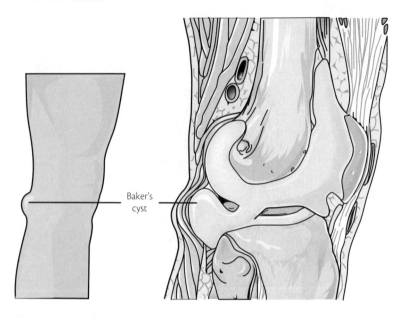

Baker's
cyst

Figure 4.2 A baker's cyst is seen as a swelling behind the knee. It forms when joint fluid collects behind the knee. The swelling may be due to inflammation or from other causes, such as arthritis.

bones that make up the spine) in the lower neck, lower chest and lower back. Osteoarthritis in any of these locations can cause pain, muscle spasms and diminished mobility.

Osteoarthritis of the spine can lead to complications. Bony outgrowths of the vertebrae in the lower spine may press on the nerves within the spinal canal, causing low back pain and pain in the legs that is worsened by exercise, and also numbness and tingling of the affected parts of the body. Osteoarthritis of the lower spine may also cause the normally aligned vertebrae to slip out of alignment.

When the spine is affected in the neck, narrowing of the spinal canal can cause damage to the spinal cord, resulting in arm or leg weakness, difficulty walking or loss of control of the bowel or bladder.

Hands

Osteoarthritis of the fingers occurs most often in older women and may be inherited within families. Osteoarthritis causes the formation of hard bony

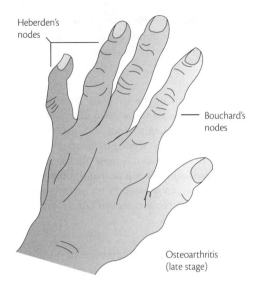

Figure 4.3 Bouchard's nodes.

enlargements (nodes) of the small joints of the fingers. The characteristic appearances of these finger nodes can be helpful in diagnosing osteoarthritis.

Osteoarthritis may cause enlargements of the last joints on the fingers (the distal interphalangeal or DIP joints) called Heberden's nodes. The bony deformity is a result of the bone and cartilage spurs (osteophytes) from the osteoarthritis in that joint. Osteoarthritis may also cause enlargements of the middle joints of the finger (the proximal interphalangeal or PIP joints) called Bouchard's nodes.

Osteoarthritis also frequently damages the base of the thumb, which may give the hand a squared appearance.

Gelatinous cysts, which sometimes go away on their own, may also form in the finger joints.

Hips

Osteoarthritis frequently strikes the weight-bearing joints in one or both hips. Pain develops slowly, usually in the groin and on the outside of the hips, or sometimes in the buttocks. The pain may also radiate to the knee, making the diagnosis less clear. Those with osteoarthritis of the hip often have a restricted range of motion (particularly when trying to rotate the hip) and walk with a limp, because they slightly turn the affected leg to avoid pain. The pain of hip osteoarthritis is often made worse during activities such as walking, getting in and out of the car and putting socks or stockings on.

Shoulder

Osteoarthritis is less common in the shoulder area than in other joints. Osteoarthritis may cause vague shoulder discomfort, bony outgrowths that irritate or even tear the surrounding tendons and, occasionally, marked pain and restriction of movement. It may develop in the shoulder joint itself (called the glenohumeral joint). In such cases it is most often associated with a previous injury, and patients gradually develop pain and stiffness in the back of the shoulder. Osteoarthritis also can develop in the joint between the shoulder blade and the collarbone, the acromioclavicular (AC) joint.

Feet

Osteoarthritis often affects the feet. Inflammation of the joint at the base of the big toe may cause a bunion or stiffness of the joint and may make it difficult to walk.

5

How is osteoarthritis diagnosed?

> ➔ **Key points**
>
> ◆ Osteoarthritis is a clinical diagnosis based on the symptoms and signs you present with.
>
> ◆ X-rays can be helpful to confirm this diagnosis and where necessary laboratory tests can help to rule out other conditions.
>
> ◆ Please seek help from a health professional to make the correct diagnosis.

There is no single sign, symptom or test result that allows a definitive diagnosis of osteoarthritis. Instead, the diagnosis is based on a consideration of several factors, including the presence of the characteristic signs and symptoms of osteoarthritis (described in the previous chapter in greater detail) and where necessary the results of X-rays and laboratory tests.

Medical history (symptoms)

A person's medical history often suggests the presence of osteoarthritis. A doctor will ask about the presence, duration and pattern of joint symptoms, and any other symptoms. A doctor will also ask about the effects of the symptoms on daily activities. The usual symptom is pain involving one or only a few joints. Joint involvement is often asymmetric – meaning that it can affect joints on either side of the body to a different extent. Morning joint stiffness that usually resolves within 30 minutes is also common. As the disease progresses, night pain, prolonged joint stiffness and joint enlargement are evident. Crepitus, a grating sensation in the joint, is a late symptom. Limitation of joint movement may be due to flexion contractures (inability to fully extend the joint) or mechanical obstructions (joint locking).

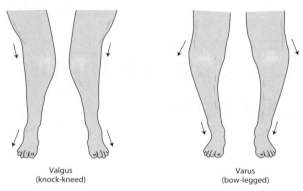

Valgus
(knock-kneed)

Varus
(bow-legged)

Figure 5.1 (a) The valgus deformity (knocked knees) showing the uneven pressure on the knee joint; (b) the varus deformity (bow-legged) showing the uneven pressure on the knee joint.

Physical examination (signs)

The signs noted during a physical exam often support a diagnosis of osteoarthritis. OA's usual expression involves multiple structures. Consequently, medical diagnosis is most appropriately based upon careful clinical examination of overall joint function. During a physical exam, a doctor will check for joint swelling, abnormalities in range of motion, tenderness and bony outgrowths. He or she will also check for changes in joint alignment and a loss of muscle mass around the joints.

Clinical examination for hip and or knee OA should include an assessment of body mass (because this risk factor is so important in predisposing to OA and increasing the rate of progression once disease is evident) and postural alignment in both standing and walking. Assessing knee alignment for the presence of genu varum (bow-legged) or genu valgum (knock-kneed) malalignment is most easily seen when the patient is asked to stand with their legs together. In the presence of genu varum, the feet will come together even while the knees remain separated, while in the presence of genu valgum the knees will touch and the feet will remain separated (Fig. 5.1).

The barefoot standing posture of the feet should also be noted so that recommendations can be made for supportive footwear. The assessment of joint range of motion, stability of the ligaments, muscle strength and tenderness to focal palpation constitutes a basic physical examination.

Clinical features that help to establish a diagnosis of symptomatic knee OA include gradually developing local knee pain and stiffness, limited active and passive motion, intra-articular (inside the joint) swelling that reoccurs with activity, crepitus, a past history of knee injury or arthroscopic (telescopic) surgery, focal tenderness over the affected regions of the medial (inside) or lateral (outside) joint margin, and advancing age. Knee OA is unusual in people younger than 40.

During the clinical examination, some attempt must be made to rule out referred pain to the knee from the hip or lumbar spine. A scanning examination can be directed to address concerns about concurrent groin, thigh or low back symptoms along with an assessment of the pain response to passive hip internal rotation. Sciatica (lumbar radiculitis) is a common cause of posterior or lateral knee pain and should be ruled out with a straight leg raise test while you are lying flat on your back. Further evaluation is indicated when the diagnosis remains uncertain, response to therapy is not as expected or significant clinical changes occur.

X-rays

X-rays are a form of electromagnetic radiation (like light); they are of higher energy, however, and can penetrate the body to form an image on film. Structures that are dense (such as bone) will appear white, air will be black, and other structures will be shades of grey depending on their density.

X-rays are often helpful for making a diagnosis of OA, although there is often a discrepancy between the severity of symptoms and the results of X-rays in people with osteoarthritis. Radiographs are not required for every person who presents with symptoms consistent with osteoarthritis. Patients whose clinical history or course suggests other conditions should undergo radiographic evaluation. This includes patients with trauma, joint pain at night, progressive joint pain (without prior radiography), significant family history of inflammatory arthritis and children younger than 18 years. Simple X-ray testing can be very helpful to exclude other causes of pain in a particular joint, as well as assisting in the decision-making as to when or if surgery should be considered.

Bearing in mind that radiographs are notoriously insensitive to the earliest features of OA, the absence of positive radiographic findings should not be interpreted as confirming the complete absence of symptomatic disease. Conversely, the presence of positive radiographic findings does not guarantee that an osteoarthritic joint is also the active source of the patient's current knee symptoms. Asymptomatic radiographic OA (presence of X-ray OA without symptoms) is common, especially among older patients in whom radiographic findings are also frequently present in multiple joints.

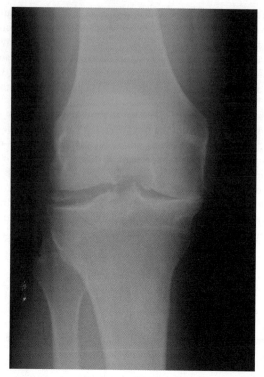

Figure 5.2 An X-ray taken from the front of the knee demonstrating narrowing of the medial (inner) joint space, increased bony whiteness (sclerosis) and osteophytes (new bone and cartilage) forming at the inner joint margin.

OA can occur in any joint of the body, but it is most common in the knees, hips, low back, fingers and at the base of the thumb. While techniques for obtaining images may vary between different regions of the body, the radiographic features of OA are similar (Fig. 5.2). The following findings on X-rays suggest the presence of osteoarthritis:

◆ Narrowing of the joint space (the space between the two bones), indicating the loss of cartilage. This provides a useful indication of the location and severity of OA, but it is not solely indicative of articular cartilage (cartilage lining the end of the bones) loss. It can also reflect changes in alignment and the meniscus.

◆ An abnormal hardening of the bone beneath the cartilage surface is termed radio-opaque thickening or sclerosis.

◆ Bony outgrowths (osteophytes) appear characteristically at the joint margins as a result of new bone and cartilage/growth.

◆ The presence of cysts beneath the surface of the bone.

◆ A film of the long limb will demonstrate the characteristic bow-legged appearance ovarus malalignment) of right knee with medial tibiofemoral OA (inner knee joint).

Laboratory tests

There is no laboratory test for the diagnosis of osteoarthritis. Laboratory tests may indirectly aid the diagnosis of osteoarthritis by helping to rule out other conditions with similar symptoms that can mimic osteoarthritis.

◆ Erythrocyte sedimentation rate (ESR) – the erythrocyte sedimentation rate does not specifically indicate osteoarthritis. A high ESR may indicate that arthritis is being caused by an inflammatory condition.

◆ Rheumatoid factor – an antibody called rheumatoid factor is present in most people with rheumatoid arthritis and can help distinguish osteoarthritis from rheumatoid arthritis.

◆ Synovial fluid analysis – small samples of synovial fluid (the fluid bathing the joint) can be withdrawn and analysed during a procedure called arthrocentesis. During arthrocentesis, a sterile needle is used to remove joint fluid for further analysis. In people with osteoarthritis, this fluid is usually clear and viscous and contains few inflammatory cells. In osteoarthritis, the white blood cell count is usually less than 500 cells per mm^2 and is composed predominantly of mononuclear cells. In cases of inflammation due to gout, infection or other forms of inflammatory arthritis, the white blood cell count is usually greater than 2,000 cells per mm^2, and the predominant cell type is usually the neutrophil (type of white cell). The presence of crystals in the fluid may be an indication of gout. Removal of joint fluid and injection of corticosteroids into the joints during arthrocentesis can help relieve pain, swelling, and inflammation.

Other investigations

When the results of other tests are inconclusive, a doctor may recommend an MRI or arthroscopy. In an arthroscopy, a thin lighted tube is moved into the joint space, allowing direct inspection of the joint structures.

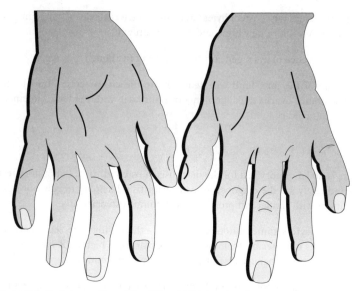

Figure 5.3 Nodular swelling of the DIP and PIP joints (small joints at the ends and middle of the fingers) of the hand consistent with osteoarthritis.

Arthroscopy is especially useful for detecting damage of cartilage, which is not visible on X-rays.

Diagnostic criteria

Formal criteria are helpful for diagnosing osteoarthritis in specific joints. These are used in the clinical setting as well as in research to increase the likelihood that a person has OA of either the knee, hand or hip. What follows are the criteria developed and proposed by the American College of Rheumatology.

◆ *Osteoarthritis of the knee.* The criteria for osteoarthritis of the knee includes the presence of knee pain plus at least three of the following:

1. Age greater than 50 years.

2. Morning stiffness lasting less than 30 minutes.

3. Crackling or grating sensation (crepitus).

4. Bony tenderness of the knee.

5. Bony enlargement of the knee.

6. No detectable warmth of the joint to the touch.

Laboratory tests and X-rays are often used in addition to these criteria to diagnose osteoarthritis of the knee.

◆ *Osteoarthritis of the hand.* The criteria for osteoarthritis of the hand includes the presence of hand pain plus at least three of the following:

1. Bony enlargement of at least two or more of ten selected joints.

2. Bony enlargements of two or more distal interphalangeal (DIP (joints at the end of the fingers)) joints.

3. Fewer than three swollen metacarpophalangeal (MCP (knuckle)) joints.

4. Deformity of at least one of the ten selected joints.

Osteoarthritis of the hand can often be diagnosed on the basis of these criteria alone, and laboratory tests and X-rays may be unnecessary.

◆ *Osteoarthritis of the hip.* The diagnosis of osteoarthritis of the hip relies on the results of laboratory tests and X-rays. The criteria for osteoarthritis of the hip include the presence of hip pain plus at least two of the following:

1. A normal erythrocyte sedimentation rate (ESR).

2. The presence of bony outgrowths (osteophytes) on X-rays.

3. The presence of narrowing in the joint space on X-rays, indicating a loss of cartilage.

Conclusion

Osteoarthritis is a clinical diagnosis based on the symptoms and signs you present with. X-rays can be helpful to confirm this diagnosis and where necessary laboratory tests can help to rule out other conditions. *Please seek help from a health professional to make the correct diagnosis and do not use this chapter for making your own diagnosis.*

6

The long-term outlook for osteoarthritis

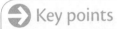

Key points

♦ Research has helped us to understand the natural course of osteo-arthritis.

♦ It is not inevitable that your osteoarthritis will get worse, it can remain stable and even improve with time.

♦ Being overweight is a strong risk factor for the worsening of osteo-arthritis and its symptoms.

♦ It is helpful to have a good understanding of factors that can cause osteoarthritis to progress to enable us to develop a management plan. This will include a number of things that can done at home without the need for medical input.

? Frequently asked questions (FAQ)

Like many other chronic conditions, people who have been diagnosed with osteoarthritis like to know what the natural course of the disease is. [Questions such as: will it deteriorate? [Will it affect every joint? [Will I need a joint replacement? are commonly asked.

In practice doctors treat patients with varying degrees of osteoarthritis: at one end of the spectrum are those with very mild symptoms and just one joint affected, whilst at the other end of the scale are those with severe progressive osteoarthritis and multiple joint involvement. The answers to these common questions are therefore not black and white, as the natural course of osteoarthritis can vary considerably between individuals.

Research and osteoarthritis progression

Research plays a vital role in helping us learn more regarding the natural progression of osteoarthritis. Over the past two to three decades there have been studies both in Europe and in America that have followed patients for periods ranging from 2 to 15 years with the aim of establishing the natural progression of osteoarthritis to see if there are any familiar patterns to the disease process. This research has examined the disease progression in the most common sites affected by osteoarthritis, the knee, the hip and the hand, and has mainly concentrated on the following signs and symptoms:

◆ The amount of pain and discomfort and the loss of function experienced.

◆ The X-ray changes that show a loss of articular cartilage, the presence of osteophytes and occasionally sclerosis of the bone.

◆ Pathological changes to the bone and cartilage structure and the other components of the joint.

Having these three main areas of focus makes the research projects more complex, especially as we already know from previous chapters that the amount of pain does not always correlate with the amount of deterioration of joint structure and vice versa.

The results of research to date has, however, identified three conclusions regarding the natural progression of OA:

1. There are some general factors that can influence the progression of OA for individuals.

2. Each joint has a different natural progression.

3. Not all joints affected by OA will progress.

General factors affecting the progression of osteoarthritis

There have been several general factors associated with the progression of OA in the joints in general. Some of them are intrinsic and others are extrinsic, that is, some are due to our genetic make up whilst others are influenced by environmental factors such as obesity, muscle weakness and injury. These factors are taken into consideration when trying to ascertain the course of OA in an individual. Fortunately it is possible to make some positive changes with some of the environmental factors mentioned below and these in turn can alter the progression of osteoarthritis.

Age

Unfortunately we are unable to stop the body clock, and the older we become the more susceptible we are to developing osteoarthritis, so much so that by the age of 75 years it is estimated 90 per cent of us will develop osteoarthritis that is visible on X-ray in at least one joint, although not all of us will develop symptoms.

Multiple joint involvement

There is good news, however. If you have osteaoarthritis of one joint you will not automatically develop osteoarthritis in your other joints, indeed many of us will know a friend or colleague who has osteoarthritis of just one joint.

However, research has demonstrated that if two or more joints are involved with osteoarthritis there is a greater risk of the disease progressing within a joint. This has been demonstrated in studies of the knee and the hip where there is more disease progression when another joint has osteoarthritis. For instance the presence of Heberden's nodes on the fingers (see Hand osteo-arthritis below) can increase the progression of knee osteoarthritis up to sixfold. This increased risk is also present if two of the same type of joint are affected, for example bilateral (both) knee osteoarthritis has been found to be more likely to progress than unilateral (one) knee osteoarthritis.

Obesity

We are already aware that being overweight is a major contribution to the ini-tial onset of osteoarthritis of the weight-bearing joints knee and hip, and also of the hand, especially in women. Research has also shown that obesity has a very strong link to the progression of osteoarthritis in these joints.

The mechanisms behind the progression of the disease in those who are over-weight is due first to excessive loading upon the joints through daily activity, which in turn causes breakdown of some cartilage and also puts huge stress on other structures of the joint; and secondly, is due to metabolic factors. In those who are overweight it is thought that abnormal cholesterol levels and glu-cose circulating in the blood and glucose circulating in the blood, along with chronic inflammation, can affect the progression of osteoarthritis: this is why, the disease develops in non-weight-bearing joints such as those on the hand.

Fortunately studies have shown that it is possible to reduce the progression of osteoarthritis by losing weight through changing diets and lifestyles, and Part 2 of this book will discuss this in more detail.

Muscle weakness and joint injury

Chapter 3 discussed the importance of muscle strength and tone in helping to maintain what is termed 'a stable joint': one that will ensure it moves in the correct direction with good power. In a good joint all the structures work together to maintain this stability. Studies have shown that previous injuries to joints and poor muscle strength are factors that can accelerate osteoarthritis progression. Unfortunately surgical correction following an injury does not completely protect the joint from osteoarthritis in the future.

Protecting our joints and muscles prior to exercising by gentle stretching and warming up and cooling down are now routinely practised in schools, colleges and at exercise classes, and will help reduce injuries that will prevent the onset of osteoarthritis of that specific joint in the long term. Muscle strength can be improved to prevent progression, and Part 2 of this book will cover it in more detail.

Specific joints and the progression of osteoarthritis

Most research to date has focused on the knee, the hip and the hand. Although other sites are discussed below, there is far less research with which to correctly identify specific natural progression.

Knee

The knee is one of the more complex joints of the musculo-skeletal system: it has three compartments all of which can develop osteoarthritis. In general, research has shown that the progression of knee osteoarthritis is often very slow, often taking years to develop and often remaining stable for several years. In a minority of people symptoms can sometimes improve after one year following diagnosis, although it is very rare for signs on X-ray to improve.

Those who have experienced a significant knee injury tend to develop osteoarthritis of this joint at an earlier age, the disease developing up to 20 years earlier than if no injury were sustained. Unfortunately the knee joint is prone to injury due to its complexity as a joint and also due to its function. In general it is thought that the rate of progression is accelerated by continued heavy weight-bearing activities and repetitive movements such as kneeling. Excess body weight also accelerates the disease process, as mentioned above.

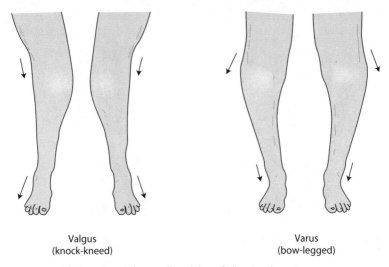

Valgus
(knock-kneed)

Varus
(bow-legged)

Figure 6.1 (a) The valgus deformity (knock-knees) showing the uneven pressure on the knee joint; (b) the varus deformity (bow-legged) showing the uneven pressure on the knee joint.

Those who have osteoarthritis with altered alignment such as valgus or varus alignment (commonly called knock-knees or bow legs), osteoarthritis experience of this joint five times more often than those who have neither abnormality. This occurs as a result of excessive uneven loading of weight within the joint progression, which leads to premature stresses on the other joint structures.

Initially the symptoms of pain and stiffness are treated with analgesics and physiotherapy, which enable normal activity levels, but as the disease progresses people experience more pain and difficulties performing daily activities such as walking, climbing stairs or climbing in and out of the bath. Over time the knee joint stiffness and swelling increases in 55 per cent of people, which often leads to less activity. Treatments at this stage include injection therapy, stronger analgesics and occasionally surgical interventions if the symptoms are resistant to other treatments.

The longer studies that followed patients for 11–15 years with X-rays have shown that between 33 to 66 per cent of subjects who have OA of the knee displayed worsening of the disease as measured by further loss of cartilage. Over the years scientists have studied X-rays to ascertain if the presence of any one specific feature such as osteophytes, sclerosis and joint space narrowing

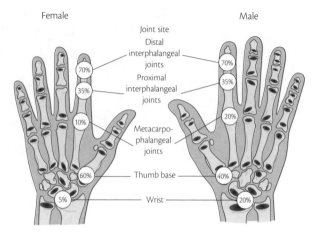

Figure 6.2 How common the involvement of each joint of the hand is for men and women with osteoarthritis of the hand.

can determine the course that the OA will take, and they concluded that all the features are important determinants of OA progression of this joint.

Hip

There has been less research into the natural course of OA of the hip joint, partly because it is thought people do not visit their clinician until they are in the late stages of the disease. However, it is suggested that the progression in this joint is more rapid and aggressive than the knee joint, often ranging from three months to three years before seeking surgery. Two studies have shown that for a small number of people the symptoms and sometimes the radiological changes can improve, but they are the minority. As the hip is a weight-bearing joint its acceleration is affected by excessive loading of weight, either through an increase in body weight or through heavy manual work. For those who have been born with congenital hip abnormalities the onset of OA in this joint starts earlier at approximately 40 years of age.

Initially the pain is controlled with analgesics and many people find using a walking stick beneficial. As the disease progresses the pain when walking increases, night-time pain can develop and up to 60 per cent of people seek surgical treatment following two years from initial diagnosis. One complication of hip OA is the death of bone tissue (osteonecrosis), which tends to occur in the late stages of its progression. This would necessitate surgery.

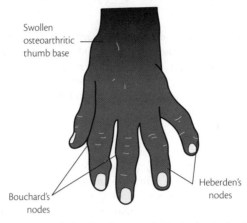

Figure 6.3 A classic picture of a hand with osteoarthritis that has Heberden's nodes and Bouchard's nodes.

Hand

OA of the hand usually affects the distal phalangeal joint (DIP) and the proximal phalangeal joint (PIP) joint of the fingers and also the base of the thumb and is common with women in their 50s. The natural history of OA in the fingers is very different than that of the knee and hip joints. It starts with a general ache in the affected joint, which comes and goes, followed by an inflammatory phase where the joints can become swollen and tender. During this phase, which often lasts one to two years, Heberden's and Bouchard's nodes develop: these are initially firm but later become hard and bony. After several years the pain and tenderness subside but the swellings become firm and fixed, resulting in reduced movement. Often during the seventh and eighth decade the symptoms in the joints settle, but the nodes and deformities usually remain. Many people are anxious regarding the appearance of these but they rarely progress to the point where a joint replacement is necessary and at this stage, despite some stiffness, are often free of pain.

The base of the thumb can also develop OA and initially becomes painful when writing or using a keyboard. As with OA of the fingers mentioned above, the symptoms are initially treated with analgesics and non-steroidal anti-inflammatory drugs. For some people OA of the thumb base necessitates splints, injections and occasionally surgery.

Shoulder

This joint is less commonly affected by OA and there has been little research into it with regard to OA progression. Often OA of the shoulder has developed as a consequence of trauma. If conservative treatment of analgesia and non-steroidal anti-inflammatory drugs fail to relieve symptoms or improve function then surgery is considered, although a full range of movement is not always achieved following this.

Foot

Although OA can occur in any joint of the foot it is the big toe joint that is most commonly affected. Wearing well-fitting shoes often relieves pain, and orthotics is also helpful for some people. Generally people manage OA in this joint using analgesics and non-steroidal anti-inflammatories, although a small proportion are referred for surgical treatment if symptoms continue to be troublesome.

Spine

Osteoarthritis of the spine is often over-diagnosed by many people who incorrectly label disc degeneration or simple mechanical back pain as being arthritic. OA of the spine only affects the facet joints and its course is one of a natural progression over many years, sometimes causing flare-ups of pain along the way. Although spinal pain is common in the general population there has been little research into the progression of facet joint OA.

Conclusion

Previous studies have shown that progression of OA varies between each type of joint and can be influenced by several factors, some of which are intrinsic while others are environmental. For these reasons the natural course of OA can vary enormously between individuals and not everyone develops widespread OA requiring surgery.

To some degree it is up to individuals and choices that they make as to how the disease progresses, and how they choose to manage it can alter the progression and symptoms of OA.

Unfortunately there is no cure at present for OA, but research continues to play a vital role in enabling us to understand the disease process in more detail, which in turn will help us to treat it effectively and slow its natural progression.

Part 2

The management of osteoarthritis

7

The management of osteoarthritis

Our intention in writing this book is to produce a patient-friendly resource that can provide the interested person who has osteoarthritis with information to help them to manage their osteoarthritis. We hope this book will expand your knowledge of OA and help with your own disease management.

Osteoarthritis is a disease of the whole joint. It can cause pain and inflammation, and stiffness that often lead to reduced function. These physical symptoms can affect us in many different ways, and have an impact on our work, our home life and on our leisure time, as well as our moods and emotions. We are all individuals and for some people with osteoarthritis everyday tasks such as washing, dressing, cooking and shopping can become difficult tasks to complete, while for others thoughts and emotions can become unhelpful. Although osteoarthritis is a disease of the joint, it can have consequences that impact greatly on our lifestyles. For this reason, when considering the management for osteoarthritis, it is important to assess each person individually so as to ensure that the areas of that person's life that are affected by osteoarthritis can be addressed.

Like other chronic diseases, there is no sole treatment or cure, instead there are several strategies to use that can help manage the condition. Similarly people who have diabetes are urged not to just take their insulin, but also to reduce weight if overweight, to have a healthy diet, to monitor their blood sugar levels and so on. All these strategies help maintain a safe blood sugar level ~ improve good health, which can reduce the risk of developing complicat' who manage patients with osteoarthritis recognize that to ma it is best to use them as part of a package and incorporate r together. For instance, do not just take pain medicine toms, but consider your weight, your fitness levels evaluate your daily patterns of activity – are you r

In America guidelines to address the treatment for osteoarthritis have been written by the American College of Rheumatology (ACR) and in Europe these guidelines have been written by the European league against Rheumatism (EULAR), using the evidence from trials and from expert advise. Although they differ slightly, the advice regarding treatment is similar. Both have these broad aims:

1. Offering information about both the disease and its management.

2. Helping to control your pain.

3. Identifying difficulties and so helping to improve function and decrease disability.

4. Altering the disease process and its consequences where possible.

The fourth of these aims, 'altering the disease process and its consequences', is aimed at altering the underlying structures in the joint that are affected in OA in order to reduce the long-term morbidity associated with osteoarthritis. Of all of the aims it is often the most difficult to achieve but the most meaningful if it can be done.

Broadly speaking, altering the disease process can be done in one of two ways:

1. The first is to modify one of the risk factors known to be associated with the progression of disease. This includes modifying risk factors such as body weight, joint alignment and muscle strength. For example, if you are overweight, losing weight will slow the progression of structural changes within your joint. If your joint is malaligned, using treatments aimed at improving alignment, such as braces or shoes, could alter long-term progression of the disease. Similarly, if you have muscle weakness or joint instability then improving muscle strength may impact on the structural course of your osteoarthritis.

2. The second is to take an agent/medication that may modify the underlying structure of your joint. At this point it is difficult to make any strong recommendations for the patient with osteoarthritis, but watch this space! There is some provisional evidence that glucosamine sulphate may fulfil this purpose.

These general aims are not in any order of importance and ideally they should all be addressed in some form. Where they are not being addressed by your health professional it is important that you arm yourself with some knowledge (such as that contained within this book) so that you can attempt to institute self-management strategies or so you can ask your caring health professional about them.

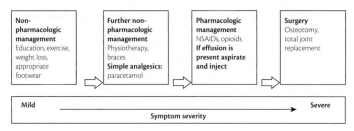

Figure 7.1 Stepwise algorithm for the management of the patient with OA. This is an example of a treatment algorithm that is modified according to your response and the clinician's preference. It highlights the encompassing need to consider non-pharmacologic management as first-line treatment for all persons with osteoarthritis before drugs and surgery. If symptoms persist or are more severe you would move along the algorithm from left to right.

What forms of treatments are available?

The forms of conventional treatment strategies that are available today include some educational groups, pain-management groups, pain-relieving medications, glucosamine sulphate, physiotherapy, injections and surgery. But what treatment should be tried first? It may not be appropriate, for instance, for people to seek a surgical opinion as the first line of treatment, as surgery is not usually indicated for most people who have osteoarthritis! With the knowledge of treatments available, clinicians may follow the steps shown in Figure 7.1. As you can see, the first stages of treatment address non-invasive treatments. For many people with osteoarthritis these two steps alone will be sufficient to manage the condition and prevent its progression and they should always be tried first before moving onto step three and four.

These treatments are discussed more fully in the following chapters of this book.

Step one: the non-medicinal approach

This includes:

◆ *Education* – OA is a chronic condition for which self-management plays a very important role. Everyone with osteoarthritis should be encouraged to participate in available self-management programmes (such as those conducted by the Arthritis Foundation). These programmes provide information regarding the natural history of your OA, and provide resources for social support and instruction on coping skills as well as reducing the anxieties that many people have when first diagnosed with osteoarthritis. They have been shown to have a meaningful and long-standing impact on osteoarthritis management for individuals with this disease. For those who do not have access to such programmes, medical centres, physiotherapists and clinicians may be able to offer leaflets and literature regarding osteoarthritis, and some physiotherapists run osteoarthritis education groups. Further information can also be obtained via the Internet (addresses are included at the back of this book). The more information you have regarding the condition, the easier it will be to manage the disease. We hope this book will be of great value here.

◆ *Weight loss* – anyone who is overweight with hip and knee OA should be encouraged to lose weight through a combination of diet and exercise. The Arthritis, Diet, and Activity Promotion trial (an 18-month study) showed that diet and exercise leads to overall improvements in self-reported measures of pain and function in older overweight and obese adults with knee OA (see Chapter 10, Weight control).

◆ *Appropriate supportive footwear* should be worn by anyone with osteoarthritis in their lower limbs. There are a number of ways in which footwear can potentially modify impact loading through the leg and thus reduce impact that potentially may lead to pain if you have OA in the knee or hip. Shoes should be supportive and have a low heel (even a heel 1.5 inches high can cause greater strain on the knee joint). Many people with knee pain gain relief with customized orthotic inserts and supportive shoes. For those with knee pain, a supportive running shoe may assist in providing needed protection and thus reducing the symptoms associated with knee OA.

Step two: further non-medicinal treatments

◆ *Exercise* increases aerobic capacity, muscle strength and endurance, and also facilitates weight loss. Quadriceps strengthening exercises have been demonstrated to lead to improvements in pain and function (see Chapter 9 Exercise, for more details).

◆ *Canes.* Perhaps the simplest way to reduce mechanical stress on a sensitive knee or hip is to use a cane. In order to provide maximal benefit, the cane should be held in the hand on the opposite side to the painful limb and put firmly to the ground with each footfall of the painful side.

Step three: medicinal therapies

◆ Simple over the counter pain relievers (analgesics). Paracetamol (Acetaminophen) is the oral analgesic of choice for mild to moderate pain in osteoarthritis. It reduces pain and is well tolerated at the recommended dose (up to 4g/day) and as such is recommended as the first analgesic to try by most physicians involved in the management of patients with osteoarthritis.

◆ Vitamins and supplements. There are a number of supplements and vitamins marketed for the treatment of osteoarthritis. The best known of these are glucosamine sulphate and chondroitin sulphate. They are generally very well-tolerated, reduce pain and may slow the progression of the OA (see Chapter 11 on the role of glucosamine for further details).

◆ Pain-relieving medicines (analgesics).

1. Non-steroidal anti-inflammatory drugs (NSAIDs) can be considered for those who respond inadequately to paracetemol. However, there are certain disadvantages in routinely using NSAIDs in OA (see Chapter 12 Medicines used in osteoarthritis).

2. Opioid analgesics are useful alternatives in patients in whom NSAIDs are not suitable, ineffective and/or poorly tolerated.

3. Formulations of NSAIDs that can be applied to the skin.

4. Other medicines include amitriptyline and capsaicin. See Chapter 12 for more on medicines used in osteoarthritis.

◆ Intra-articular injections. This is an injection into the joint, and it can lead to considerable relief of pain in joints with osteoarthritis. There are two different types of injections, corticosteroids and hyaluronans – they are both effective but are used in different clinical situations. They need to be administered by a clinician and should be discussed with your doctor. (See Chapter 13 Injection therapies for more details.)

Step four: surgery

Surgery should be resisted when symptoms can be managed by the treatments mentioned in steps one, two and three. The typical indications for surgery are debilitating pain and major limitation of functions such as walking and daily activities, or impaired ability to sleep or work. Different surgical interventions include:

- ◆ Arthroscopic debridement and lavage (telescopic scraping and washout).

- ◆ Osteotomy (realigning the joint).

- ◆ Joint replacement (see Chapter 17 for further details).

Future treatments for osteoarthritis

The reason for developing OA appears to be the result of a complex interplay between mechanical (increased pressure on selected parts of the joint), cellular (related to cells) and biochemical forces. Of these factors, the mechanical forces are paramount. Although osteoarthritis is a condition associated with getting old, it should not be assumed that we can do little about its occurrence. In the field of osteoarthritis, clinicians and scientists are working hard to learn more about the disease process so as to improve treatments, prevent progression and also the onset.

Given the strong evidence for mechanical forces playing such a prominent role in the development of osteoarthritis (see Fig. 7.2) there have been few therapies to date developed to address this issue. Drug-based treatments to date have focused on reducing inflammation (e.g. non-steroidal anti-inflammatory drugs), stimulating cartilage cell (chondrocyte) function and replenishing the lubricant that is usually lacking in the joint with osteoarthritis (hyaluronans). It could be argued that unless the extra forces on the joint are not addressed then the medicines will be limited in their effectiveness.

Knee braces and orthotics

Despite knowing for many years that altering loads in individuals with knee OA is effective at relieving symptoms, use of therapies based on this principle are limited. Although they are both effective and safe, knee braces (see Fig. 7.3) are not commonly prescribed in the management of knee osteoarthritis, and when they are, their use declines rapidly with time. Knee OA is a chronic disease which requires long-term therapy, and whilst brace use has demonstrated improvement in symptoms of pain and function in short-term studies (none longer than six months), there have been no long-term controlled studies that have evaluated brace efficacy or adherence. Further longer-term studies are needed, ideally with newer brace designs that are less cumbersome and bulky and thus easier to use continually.

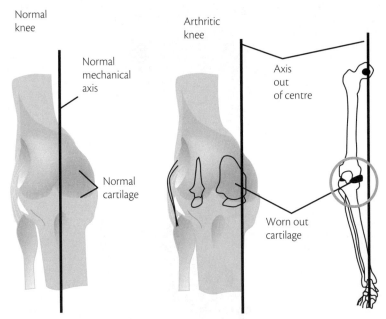

Normal knee

Normal mechanical axis

Normal cartilage

Arthritic knee

Axis out of centre

Worn out cartilage

Figure 7.2 The mechanical axis of the knee is a line extending from the centre of the hip joint to the middle of the ankle joint. This line is practically perpendicular to the ground. In a healthy, well-aligned knee joint, the axis passes closer to the middle of the knee. This allows the stresses on the knee-joint surfaces to be more uniform in all areas of the joint and well balanced. In OA, the mechanical axis is often is disturbed. This disturbance results in the overload of particular areas of the knee joint, and leads to their damage.

Tissue engineering

Another area that demonstrates great potential but again needs further research work to support its use before widespread use in people with OA is tissue engineering (see Fig. 7.4). Tissue engineering, a term that was coined in 1986, describes the science of replacing, repairing or regenerating organs or tissue. (The term is often used interchangeably with regenerative medicine.) In the field of osteoarthritis management, this includes the use of growth factors to regenerate cartilage and bone, using new technologies to enhance the healing of menisci (disc of cartilage in the knee) and ligaments, efforts to produce tissue-engineered cartilage, and the possibility of using stem cells derived from muscle or fat to improve cartilage or bone healing. These advances could, in the future, provide better treatment alternatives that may be termed biologic replacement. At the

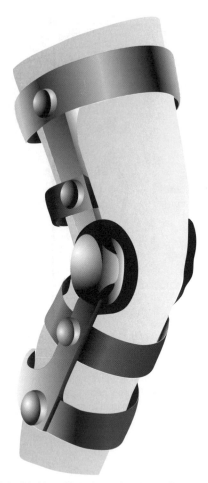

Figure 7.3 A typical double-hinged knee brace for a knee affected by osteoarthritis.

moment one of the major limitations is that unless the mechanics of the joint are also addressed these have little opportunity of success.

Obesity – a concern for the future

From a public health perspective, we could prevent approximately 50 per cent of OA if we were able to stop the obesity epidemic. Measures to control weight are essential if we are to make any public health impact on the prevalence of this burdensome disease.

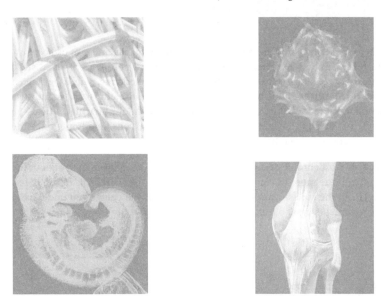

Figure 7.4 Approaches to tissue engineering include using biomaterials (scaffolds) to hold and recruit cells and promote regeneration. Cells can also be used to form tissues. Finally, growth factors (typically involved in the development of the joint) can also be used to facilitate tissue regeneration.

Altering the disease process

Several pharmacological agents, including doxycycline and diacerein, have demonstrated their ability to modify structure but are unlikely to be widely used for osteoarthritis for a number of different reasons, including costs, side-effects and relatively limited benefit. Glucosamine and chondroitin sulphate may also modify structure within the joint and are already in common use. However, many major pharmaceutical and biotechnology companies have products in their development pipeline that are intended to alter the disease process. As yet their effectiveness remains to be proved.

Greater attention to the important role of mechanical factors in OA development is required if we are to find ways of reducing the public health impact of this condition. Further research investigating weight-reduction strategies, mechanical therapies such as braces and tissue engineering are greatly needed. In time it may become apparent that rational treatment is a combination of these interventions.

Conclusion

There are several strategies that are helpful in the management of osteoarthritis. Some of the interventions are conservative and non-invasive, as in steps one and two, and can be successful for mild to moderate pain experienced with osteoarthritis. Only when these more conservative efforts fail to improve function or reduce pain to an acceptable level should pharmaceuticals be offered in steps three and four. Surgery should be considered only once the other steps have been tried.

As with most chronic diseases, the more information the person has about the condition the more in control they feel. We hope that Part 1 of this book has explained the mechanisms of osteoarthritis which will enable you understand the treatments available and how they can be helpful.

 Patient's perspective

Mrs V was a 67-year-old married woman who lived at home with her husband of 40 years. They had thee children and six grandchildren whom they adored. When Mrs V was younger she worked at the railway station as a clerk riding to and from her place of work by bicycle for 15 years until she had a fall: after this she caught the bus.

Life had always been very busy as it often is with a large family, but it had been a happy and joyous time. In her spare time Mrs V was a keen tennis player and enjoyed walking holidays with her family. At home she was the one in charge of the household. Housework was always top of her agenda as she could not abide an untidy home. Her mother too had been very houseproud, and was known for washing the kitchen floor twice a day!

Mrs V retired from the railway at the age of 60 and was looking forward to her retirement with her husband, who was in good health. Mrs V too was in good health, although for the past few years had developed some intermittent pain and stiffness in the fingers which she put down to 'all that housework'. They had made many plans on paper as to how to spend their time together which was to include a holiday to see the Swiss Alps, play at the tennis club, help with the grandchildren, join the local art club, lots of gardening and of course walking the dog on long forest walks. Life was going to be enjoyed and full of activity.

Unfortunately not long after her last day at work, she developed some knee pain when she was walking the dog round the forest. Initially she thought nothing of it, believing that it would go away: after a day or two of not walking the dog the pain did seem to settle until she came to walk the dog again and it reoccurred. This time the pain did not seem to ease and continued to cause pain when walking to the shops and around the home. The pain was reduced during the night, but on getting out of the bed in the morning it was very stiff, although this stiffness eased once she was out of the shower and having breakfast.

The pain was like a dull ache in nature and was always worse when weight-bearing as opposed to sitting down. The pain was mainly concentrated round her right knee although the thigh also ached. To help it Mrs V rubbed it and covered it with a blanket when at home to keep it warm. Her daughter suggested that she took some paracetamol but Mrs V was never keen on taking any tablets, especially for more than one day, and declined. Her husband thought she should visit the doctor – Mrs V did not like going to see doctors – 'it will get better' she told everyone.

She found that the pain did not improve although she did have good and bad spells. Over the next couple of weeks she stopped walking the dog for fear of aggravating the pain. Her husband started to do some of the chores at home so that she could rest her knee. Mrs V was now worried at what was happening, her husband was now taking over her role at home and had started to drive her everywhere. She was now missing her friends from work and was beginning to feel a little isolated and dependent on her husband, and thought 'this was not how things were meant to be in my retirement'. The pain was unpleasant, and her husband and daughters had noticed a change in her mood. She was snappy and did not seem to look forward to seeing the grandchildren at the weekend. Worst of all, the knee looked fine to her friends and they thought she might just be exaggerating the pain.

After a few weeks from the onset of the pain she visited the doctor. Following an examination of her knee and listening to the history of the pain onset he suggested that she may have osteoarthritis of the knee. He also noted that she had some osteoarthritis of the fingers also. He suggested that she tried some non-steroidal anti-inflammatories (NSAIDs) in the first instance to address the pain, and wanted to review her in two weeks.

The pain did improve a little and walking became a little easier, but it was still present. The doctor was not keen for Mrs V to continue with the NSAIDs long term due to their unwanted side-effects and suggested that she tried paracetamol on a regular basis. He gave her some literature provided by the Arthritis and Rheumatism Council (ARC) and referred her on to a physiotherapist.

The literature was very interesting and Mrs V showed it to her daughters. They used some of the websites suggested for further information. Although Mrs V did not want to have osteoarthritis she was somewhat relieved to hear from the physiotherapist that she would not end up in a wheelchair and that she would be able to walk her dogs, albeit in moderation.

The physiotherapist explained the importance of good muscle strength, and talked about some ways of achieving this that she could do at home. They also discussed how to manage her daily routines to ensure that she achieved things that were important to her. She realized that over the past few years of relying on busses and cars she had gained some unwanted and unhelpful weight, especially in the past two to three months when she missed walking the dog. She discussed with her daughter how to lose weight and about glucosamine sulphate. Her mood lifted with all the treatments she could do for herself.

Ten years later Mrs V feels the pain is well managed. She still feels in control at home, having learnt to pace herself. Tennis is not so easy, but she managed to get involved as the club secretary and has also taken up bowls (which is a slower sport). She continues to keep a check on her weight, and now that her husband has diabetes they share a healthy diet. Her grandchildren enjoyed taking Nanny shopping for some sneakers (for dog walking) and heels are only worn at weddings. Her hand pain has now settled, although she does have some nodules on some of the fingers. Some rings are now difficult to get on and off and decorating cakes is not quite as easy, but the grandchildren now enjoy doing their own. Occasionally Mrs V gets a slight ache in her left knee, but this time she is not panicking. She has learnt that there are many things that she can do herself to ensure that the osteoarthritis does not take over her life.

8

Which health professionals are involved in osteoarthritis management?

Making the most of your healthcare team

> ### Key points
>
> ♦ A well-rounded healthcare plan requires a well-rounded healthcare team.
>
> ♦ Learning to manage and being involved and educated about the therapies available will greatly enhance the improvements in pain and function you may obtain.
>
> ♦ Allowing others to assist you in managing your condition will greatly enhance the effect of your own self-management strategies.

A chronic illness affects all aspects of your life – physical, emotional, mental and even spiritual. So it's no surprise that managing the effects of your osteoarthritis means more than taking pills or doing a fitness routine. Living well with OA includes pain and function control through a variety of means – everything from exercise, eating well, weight management, taking medication, to relaxation or surgery. Having a well-rounded healthcare plan requires a well-rounded healthcare team. What follows is a compilation of some of the types of healthcare professionals that may be able to assist you in some way with helping you to manage your OA and its impact in your life. Learning to manage and being involved and educated about the therapies available will greatly enhance the improvements in pain and function you may obtain. However, central to this idea is that you have to be willing to allow others to assist you in managing your condition – this is very important. I have provided more details about those professionals who you are more likely to interact with in managing OA. As is often the case when with lists like this, one cannot be comprehensive – there may be other health professionals available who promote their expertise in managing OA.

The general practitioner/primary care physician

- ◆ *What they do for you.* General practitioners (GPs) and primary care physicians (PCPs) take care of many of your routine medical needs – checking your blood pressure, cholesterol level and heart rate. They will also monitor the medicines you use and keep track of which specialists you see.

- ◆ *What else you should know.* Your GP can handle much of your routine medical osteoarthritis-related care. They can also refer you to an appropriate specialist for further evaluation. It is essential that you have a communicative relationship with your doctor so that together you can optimize the management of your OA.

The rheumatologist

- ◆ *What they do for you.* A rheumatologist is a physician who is qualified by additional training and experience in the diagnosis and treatment of OA and other diseases of the joints, muscles and bones. In addition to treating OA, rheumatologists also treat certain autoimmune diseases, musculo-skeletal pain disorders and osteoporosis.

- ◆ *What else you should know.* A rheumatologist can provide ongoing care for your OA or act as a consultant as you continue to work with your GP/ PCP or other specialists. The role the rheumatologist plays in healthcare depends on several factors and needs. Typically the rheumatologist works with other doctors, sometimes acting as a consultant about a treatment plan. In other situations, the rheumatologist acts as a manager, relying upon the help of many skilled professionals including nurses, physiotherapists, occupational therapists, psychologists and social workers. Teamwork is important, because OA management is chronic and more often than not one management technique alone is not sufficient to control your symptoms. Healthcare professionals can help people with OA and their families cope with the changes this can cause in their lives.

The orthopaedic surgeon

♦ *What they do for you.* Orthopaedic surgeons evaluate and treat bone, joint, tendon and ligament disorders and diseases. Some specialize in particular types of surgery such as joint replacement or arthroscopy. Another doctor may refer you to an orthopaedic surgeon to determine if you are a candidate for surgery. See Chapter 17 on the different surgical options available for OA and whether or not you may be a candidate.

♦ *What else you should know.* Please recognize that surgery is not the first line of treatment for OA and should generally only be recommended once other more conservative modes of treatment have been tried and not proved helpful.

The physiotherapist/physical therapist

A physiotherapist's aim is to help people resume an active and independent life both at home and work. They will discuss patients' treatment with consultants and GPs and keep them fully informed. They will also work closely with other health professionals such as nurses and occupational therapists. Essentially, however, physiotherapists are independent practitioners who are professionally and legally responsible for their own actions.

Your first appointment

During your first appointment – which could last up to 45 minutes – you will be asked a number of questions relating to your OA. The physiotherapist will then examine you in order to find out what causes your particular difficulties. After examining you, the physiotherapist will suggest the treatment most appropriate for you, which will probably start at the following appointment.

They will also discuss the type, frequency and likely duration of your treatment. Alternatively, a self-help programme to be carried out at home may be suggested. To make it easier to examine and treat you properly, you may

71

be asked to undress down to your underwear. The physiotherapist might also advise you to bring other clothes (such as shorts or jogging pants) on subsequent visits.

Treatment

Treatment may take place in a clinic, the hospital ward, the outpatient department, a hydrotherapy pool, day hospital, school, your home or workplace. Depending on your particular needs, any of the following types of treatment may be used:

◆ *Mobilizing, stretching or strengthening exercises.* Many people with OA find that their joints become stiffer than normal. Also, some muscles may become weak with disuse. You might be shown exercises to improve the movement in your joints and others to strengthen the supporting muscles. For example, if you have knee OA the exercises will often focus on your quadriceps and hamstring muscles (muscles in the thigh).

◆ *Hydrotherapy.* Some people with OA find it is easier to move in water (hydrotherapy). Here patients can perform an exercise programme and improve their general mobility. Many people find the feeling of warmth and weightlessness allows them to move with less effort and as a result it relaxes their joints and muscles. If you have OA involving joints in your lower limbs (especially the knees or hips) this is especially useful.

◆ *Electrotherapy.* Different types of machines are used to speed up the healing process and relieve pain; some provide gentle heat to the affected joints.

◆ *Cold therapy.* When an icepack is placed on a painful joint, it can bring considerable relief. Icepacks not only increase the circulation and speed up healing, they also reduce local inflammation and relieve pain.

◆ *Relaxation.* Stress and muscle tension can make OA seem worse and learning to release this tension helps a great deal. But there is more to relaxation than simply putting your feet up. Learning effective relaxation practices can relieve mental and physical tension as well as improving your general sense of well-being.

◆ *Walking training.* This may be particularly important if your problems have caused you to walk awkwardly, especially if you now need a shoe insert, assistive device (brace) or a walking aid. The physiotherapist can advise you on the best kind of footwear and make recommendations if any adaptations (like inserts) should be fitted.

♦ *Group sessions.* You may also be asked to join exercise sessions with other people who have similar problems to your own. This is not only valuable in showing you the exercises to continue at home, but also provides you with the opportunity to meet and talk with other people who have similar difficulties.

Whichever treatment is recommended, the physiotherapist's aim will be to improve your immediate problems and to provide you with the skills, techniques and knowledge to help you cope by yourself in the long term. Often this will include continuing to do exercises at home. If this is recommended to you, do your best to continue the exercises – the improvements that you get in muscle strength are reflected in improvements in pain and function. Importantly these improvements are related to the frequency and intensity with which you continue to exercise.

Remember, it is your body, so do not be afraid to ask questions at any time during the course of your examination and treatment – especially if you are doing something that hurts. Physiotherapists are usually very happy to explain any aspect of their treatment.

The occupational therapist

♦ *Where do I see an occupational therapist?* Occupational therapists (or OTs as they are known) are usually based in hospitals. You will see a hospital-based OT after you have been given a referral from another doctor such as a rheumatologist. The OT will usually see you in the occupational therapy department, on the ward or in the outpatient clinic – although a home visit can be made.

♦ *How do I prepare for an OT appointment?* When you see an OT you will be asked about any problems you may be having. It may help to write them down before you go. Think about activities such as washing and dressing, driving your car, getting around your home, or getting up from a chair. Be sure also to mention any difficulties you may have doing your job. Make a note of any questions you want to ask. The OT will make an assessment of your condition, including which joints are affected, where there is pain and so on. Having discovered which activities are important to you and the particular problems you are experiencing, the OT will explore possible solutions with you. If necessary, this might involve advice on how best to protect the joints affected by your OA.

An occupational therapist can help:

♦ *By giving practical advice on how you can overcome everyday problems.* You may need to rethink the way you do things and this may involve using special equipment. The OT will help you choose which equipment suits your needs. Some items are easily available, such as a seat raise for your toilet that makes it easier for you to get up from the seated position. Something like a motorized scooter, or a bath lift, comes from more specialist sources.

♦ *By discussing your condition, how it affects you and what you can do to help yourself.* If you have OA you need to know how to look after vulnerable joints or so-called joint protection (reducing the load on joints that are affected). If you feel tired you can learn to make the most of your energy. You may also have other practical difficulties (such as climbing stairs, getting in and out of a car, putting your shoes and socks on, gardening or in the workplace) and questions about dealing with your limitations of function on a daily basis.

♦ *By teaching you activities to help improve strength or movement.* This may involve you coming for treatment as an outpatient, and is usually combined with physiotherapy. The aim is to improve the function of your joints. It may mean discussing activities you can do to help yourself at home.

♦ *By teaching techniques to help you cope with pain.* These may be very simple ideas which you can use at home, for instance placing a bag of frozen peas on a painful joint or wrapping a warm towel around a stiff joint. You may also be taught relaxation methods.

The pharmacist

♦ *What they do for you.* Pharmacists fill prescriptions. They help you avoid potential drug interactions and suggest strategies to avoid side-effects and improve medication use. They evaluate your medications and answer questions about them. Pharmacists can also give information about over-the-counter medications, herbal and dietary supplements.

♦ *What else you should know.* While you may see several doctors, experts suggest you stick with one pharmacist, who can then keep track of your medications and provide advice about potential problems. Taking many different types of drugs from different pharmacists increases your risk of having an adverse reaction to one of the drugs or an interaction between drugs.

The nurse

♦ *What they do for you.* In addition to taking your blood pressure, drawing blood samples and providing other routine care, nurses function as patient educators and advocates. They may talk to you about side-effects of medications, exercise and diet, and provide appropriate literature on these topics. Your nurse may serve as a liaison between you and your doctor: someone who can 'translate' a difficult-to-understand diagnosis or treatment recommendation.

♦ *What else you should know.* A 'nurse practitioner' may be part of your healthcare team. This is a nurse who has an advanced degree and is qualified to interpret lab tests and prescribe medications for you.

The mental health professional/psychologist

♦ *What they do for you.* Mental health professionals, such as psychologists, help you cope with the emotional repercussions of chronic illness such as depression, anxiety, anger or relationship problems. They may 'prescribe' anything from antidepressants to support groups. A mental health professional typically addresses these issues in one-on-one therapy sessions and helps you manage pain and stress through relaxation, meditation, hypnosis or biofeedback.

♦ *What else you should know.* OA can cause chronic pain and this can often be linked to, and exacerbated by, depression – don't ignore this possibility, and please seek help if you are feeling depressed. Most mental health professionals can refer patients to a psychiatrist for antidepressants or other medications, when appropriate.

The exercise therapist

♦ *What they do for you.* Exercise therapists are specialists in the prescription of exercise, supervising your exercise and assessing your fitness or suitability for exercise. They often complement the exercises that are given by a physical therapist, and assist and encourage you to maintain the exercise programme longer term.

♦ *What else should you know.* When starting out with exercises please be careful to ensure you don't injure yourself. Exercises should always be done in a careful and controlled manner. Some mild residual discomfort around your affected joint during and after exercise is to be expected – more often than not this simply means that you are working the area.

The nutritionist/dietician

♦   *What they do for you.* The nutritionist/dietician can advise you about getting adequate nutrition and also managing your weight. For OA it is important that you are getting adequate vitamin D and also omega 3 fatty acids. In addition excess weight can exacerbate your symptoms of OA and only through weight reduction (preferably through a combination of calorie restriction and exercise) can you manage this problem and achieve result-ant improvements in your pain and function.

♦   *What else should you know.* With your dietician set realistic targets. Aim for these and importantly maintain them. Changing life-long habits can be hard, but finding alternatives to eating unhealthy snacks can make an enormous difference.

The podiatrist

♦   *What they do for you.* Podiatrists treat conditions affecting your foot or ankle, are licensed to perform surgery and prescribe medication. They focus on controlling inflammation, preserving joint function and treating diseases or abnormalities (bunions, corns, calluses, etc.).

♦   *What else you should know.* Most podiatrists also focus on preventing foot problems that may occur due to your foot's shape or abnormalities. In OA the alignment or posture of your foot can contribute to loading at the knee or hip. Podiatrists can assist in providing advice about footwear and if necessary prescribe orthotics (shoe inserts).

The physiatrist/rehabilitation physician

♦   *What they do for you.* Physical medicine and rehabilitation (PMandR) or physiatry is a branch of medicine dealing with functional restoration of a person affected by physical disability. Physical medicine and rehabilita-tion involves the management of disorders that alter the function and performance of the patient. Emphasis is placed on the optimization of function through the combined use of medications, physical modalities (such as exercise), and experiential training approaches.

The osteopath

* *What they do for you.* Practitioners of osteopathy, called osteopaths (or osteopathic physicians in the US), have a holistic approach: osteopathic philosophy requires addressing the whole person in diagnosis, prevention and treatment of illness, disease and injury, using manual and physical therapies.

* *What else you should know.* In the USA, physical or manual treatment carried out by D.O.s (Doctor of Osteopathic Medicine) is referred to as Osteopathic Manual Medicine or Osteopathic Manipulative Medicine (both abbreviated OMM). In other countries, manual treatment by osteopaths is simply referred to as osteopathic treatment, similar to chiropractic, although the distinction between the two professions remains important to both.

The goal of OMM is the resolution of somatic dysfunction (impaired or altered function of musculoskeletal system) to reestablish the self-regulatory mechanisms of the body. There are various techniques applied to the musculo-skeletal system as OMM. These are normally employed together with dietary, postural, and occupational advice, as well as counselling to help patients recover from illness and injury, and to minimize pain and disease. Most osteopaths view manual therapies as a complement to physiotherapy, and the judicious use of invasive therapies (pharmaceuticals and surgery) where necessary.

The clergy

* *What they do for you.* A religious leader can assist you with your spiritual needs. They will pray with or for you, direct you to appropriate religious texts and provide spiritual guidance such as counselling or referrals to other services.

* *What else you should know.* Many religious leaders are trained in counselling and are frequently consulted in lieu of a mental healthcare professional.

The chiropractor

* *What they do for you.* Chiropractors help relieve pain and increase your range of motion through manual manipulation of joints.

* *What else you should know.* Chiropractors focus on natural healthcare treatments, and do not perform surgery or prescribe medicine. They are trained, however, to diagnose conditions that would require treatment by a medical doctor – and refer patients to the proper healthcare provider.

The acupuncturist

- *What they do for you.* Acupuncturists help to relieve pain by inserting small needles into certain areas of the body. According to research acupuncture may cause the release of endorphins, or painkilling hormones, and has been shown to be a helpful adjunct to other treatments in managing pain in OA.

- *What else you should know.* Some professional acupuncturists may be doctors, but most typically are not. Based upon a 2000-year-old system rooted in Chinese philosophy, acupuncture involves inserting fine needles into specific points in the body, though it is rarely painful. It seems to relieve pain by diverting or changing the painful sensations which are sent to the brain from damaged tissues and also by stimulating the body's own painkillers (the so-called endorphins and encephalins). This painkilling effect may only last a short time at the beginning, but repeated treatment (usually about six or eight weekly sessions) can bring long-term benefit, often over a period of six to nine months. If the pain returns, then some more acupuncture may help for another few months. If after a number of treatments you have not noticed any improvement don't continue with the treatment.

  As with all treatments to relieve pain (such as physiotherapy and painkilling drugs), breaking the 'pain cycle' sometimes gives long-standing relief. To some extent this depends on the stage of your OA, although acupuncture can help at almost any stage of the illness. As with many conventional treatments, it cannot cure or reverse the process of OA. Acupuncture may help someone who cannot tolerate drugs through a painful episode, or it may be used to manage pain on a long-term basis.

The social worker

- *What they do for you.* Social workers help you find the practical solutions required for convalescence or life changes such as relocating, changing jobs or caring for an ill parent. For example, if you're moving from home to an assisted living centre, a social worker can refer you to appropriate community resources. If you're planning for the care of a spouse or parent, a social worker can also refer you to in-home care services.

- *What else you should know.* Social workers also provide counselling services for people with a chronic illness.

9

Exercise

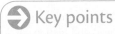 Key points

- Research has shown that participating in a regular exercise programme is a great way to feel better and move more comfortably.

- The benefit you gain will match the effort you put in.

- Optimally you should engage in a broad range of activities that suit you and your lifestyle.

Regular, moderate exercise offers a whole host of benefits to people with osteoarthritis, including stimulating the cartilage and other tissues of the joint, and building strong muscles around the joint and through this can reduce stiffness, pain and swelling. Regular physical activity also has long-term effects on your well-being. It helps promote overall health and fitness, which gives you more energy, helps you sleep better, controls your weight, assists in alleviating depression and improves your self-esteem.

Improvements in mood and well-being have been reported by regular exercisers with most types of exercise. Baseline levels of anxiety are lower in individuals who exercise regularly as compared with sedentary adults. Exercise appears to be a potent stress reducer as well. In at least one major clinical trial in the US sponsored by the National Institutes of Health, exercise and group counselling are being tested as a primary treatment for mild depression. Because depression is a concern for individuals with osteoarthritis, physical activity is therefore an important psychological adjunct to treatment. Lastly, exercise can also help stave off other health problems such as osteoporosis, diabetes and heart disease.

An exercise programme: general guidelines

What types of exercise are most suitable for someone with osteoarthritis?

The best type of exercise programme for you will depend on which joints are affected and the severity of involvement. You should seek professional advice from an expert who can devise a programme that caters for your specific needs. This should include a variety of options that you can follow, depending on the location and severity of your osteoarthritis. It should also take into consideration what type of activities appeal to you, so that you are motivated to do it regularly. There is a broad range of activities that are considered appropriate exercise for people with osteoarthritis and the best of these are:

◆ Range-of-motion (ROM) exercises (e.g. cycling, dance): these will help maintain normal joint movement and relieve stiffness, and help maintain or increase flexibility. Individuals with osteoarthritis often have a limited range of motion, especially in their lower extremity joints such as the knees or hips. Decreased range of motion associated with knee and hip OA is associated with pain, loss of function, physical limitations and an increased risk of injury and falls. In addition, to receive adequate nutrition cartilage requires regular compression and decompression to stimulate remodelling and repair. Ideally a daily exercise plan should include range-of-motion exercises and these should be specified by an exercise professional – not just 'a stretch every day' – because affected joints that are lax are easily overstretched and more vulnerable to injury.

◆ Water aerobics: aquatic aerobic training programmes that are offered in therapeutic pools are one of the best forms of exercise. Aquatic exercise has over the years been known as pool therapy, hydrotherapy, and sometimes in earlier literature even balneotherapy (spa therapy) (Bartels 2006). The treatment has to take part in water and involve exercises. Pools that are designed for people with arthritis are often kept at much warmer temperatures than recreational pools and may have specialized access ramps to make entrance to the pool easier. When the warm-water element is included, it is thought that it gives those with osteoarthritis decreased pain sensation, reduced stiffness, and causes muscle relaxation. Warm water treatment may therefore be a better base on which to start training of osteoarthritis patients than a similar training on land. This type of exercise helps to maintain range of motion of joints and also aerobic fitness. For someone with pain in the knees or hips that is related to bearing weight on the joint, exercise on land can often be painful. In contrast exercising in water, where your body weight is partly supported, can greatly enhance your ability to exercise without this discomfort.

◆ Strengthening exercises (e.g. weight-training): these help keep or increase muscle strength so the muscles are strong enough to support and protect joints affected by arthritis. The best type of strengthening programme is one that takes into account personal preferences, the type of arthritis involved and the severity of the inflammation. Strength training can be done with small free weights, exercise machines, isometrics, elastic bands and resistive water exercises. Correct positioning is critical because, if done incorrectly, strengthening exercises can cause muscle tears or more joint pain. In order to maximize the effectiveness of strengthening exercise it is necessary to combine strengthening exercises with a more complete exercise programme including ROM, stretching, functional balance and aerobic exercises.

◆ Aerobic or endurance exercises (e.g. bicycle riding, walking): these improve cardiovascular fitness, help control weight and enhance general health and well-being. Weight control can be important for people who have arthritis because extra weight puts extra pressure on many joints. It is important that this type of exercise is not high in impact (such as the heavy pounding of road running) because the pressure on affected joints can have deleterious effects. Many health clubs, swimming pools and community centres offer exercise programmes for people with physical limitations that include walking, running, cycling, aquatics and aerobic dance.

🛈 Participants in aerobic programmes have reported the following improvements:

1. increased aerobic capacity

2. decreased depression and anxiety

3. increased physical activity

4. decreased fatigue

5. increased muscular strength and flexibility

6. decreased pain

7. increased functional status.

(Brosseau 2006)

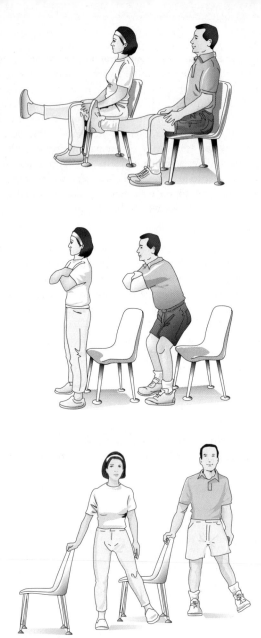

Figure 9.1 Some of the exercises that are used for persons with knee OA include knee extension, modified squat, and side lift.

It was also found that these benefits were achieved without an increase in pain or further aggravation of osteoarthritic symptoms. Interestingly enough, these findings conflict with earlier beliefs that repetitive motion causes further injury.

◆ Recreational/lifestyle activities: any recreational, or lifestyle, activity of moderate intensity, such as gardening or walking, is an important form of exercise, and does not need to be undertaken in a single session. For example, according to research, the benefits from three 10-minute walks or one 30-minute walk are similar. Current health guidelines recommend that people of all ages strive to do 30 minutes of moderate intensity lifestyle activities throughout the day on most days of the week.

Examples of moderate-intensity lifestyle activities include walking, raking leaves, gardening – even simply using the stairs.

For people with osteoarthritis, lifestyle activities, rather than traditional vigorous types of exercise, may be especially appropriate for several reasons: first, short bouts of exercise (as opposed to one continuous session) may reduce pain and prevent injury; second, intermittent episodes of activity allow individuals with arthritis more flexibility in alternating physical activity with rest; third, they provide a means by which a person who has been sedentary for a while can begin and feel able to do an exercise programme.

How does a person with osteoarthritis start an exercise programme?

Starting an exercise programme can seem like a daunting proposition. The two important things to remember are: (1) start slowly, and (2) make it fun.

People with osteoarthritis should discuss exercise options with their doctors and other healthcare providers. Many people with osteoarthritis begin with easy, range-of-motion exercises, aquatic exercise or low-impact aerobics. People with osteoarthritis can participate in a variety of, but not all, sports and exercise programmes. The doctor will know which, if any, sports are off limits. They may have suggestions about what programmes are available locally and how to get started, or they may refer the patient to a physiotherapist or exercise therapist. The therapist will design an appropriate home exercise programme and teach clients about pain-relief methods, proper body mechanics (placement of the body for a given task, such as lifting a heavy box), joint protection and how to conserve energy.

Here are some step-by-step guidelines to follow:

◆ Apply heat to sore joints (optional) – many people with osteoarthritis start their exercise programme this way.

◆   Stretch and warm up with range-of-motion exercises.

◆   Start strengthening exercises slowly with small weights (a 1- or 2-kg weight can make a big difference).

◆   Progress slowly.

◆   Use cold packs after exercising (optional) – many people with osteoarthritis complete their exercise routine this way.

◆   Add aerobic exercises.

◆   Consider appropriate recreational exercise (after doing range-of-motion, strengthening and aerobic exercises). Fewer injuries to joints affected by osteoarthritis occur during recreational exercise if it is preceded by range of motion, strengthening and aerobic exercises.

IMPORTANT NOTE: Ease off if your joints become painful.

Important exercise guidelines for a person with osteoarthritis

The three important concepts that you need to remember at all times are:

1. Begin slowly and progress gradually: the hallmark of a safe exercise pro-gramme is gradual progression in exercise intensity, complexity of move-ments and duration. Often people with osteoarthritis have lower levels of fitness due to pain, stiffness or biomechanical abnormalities (gait and alignment) that may have led to periods of immobility. Beginning with a few minutes of activity, and alternating activity with rest, should be one the initial goals.

2. Avoid rapid or repetitive movements of affected joints: Special emphasis should be placed on joint protection strategies and avoidance of activi-ties that require rapid repetitions of a movement or those that are highly percussive (abrupt) in nature. Because faster walking speeds increase joint stress, walking speed should be appropriate. Special attention must be paid to joints that are unstable. Control of shock absorption through shoe selection or use of orthotics (inserts) may be necessary.

3. Ensure the physical activity is appropriate to your needs: affected joints may be unstable and restricted in range of motion by pain, stiffness, swell-ing, bone changes or fibrosis. These joints are at higher risk for injury and care must be taken to ensure that appropriate joint protection measures

are in place. Joint protection means not placing undue stress on the joints affected by your arthritis. Activities that involve high impact, such as running, may exacerbate osteoarthritis in the knees and hips. In this instance try low-impact exercise such as water aerobics or cycling.

What pain-relief can you use during exercise?

Temporary pain relief can make it easier for people who have arthritis to exercise. Your doctor or physiotherapist can suggest a method that is best for you. The following methods have worked for many people:

◆ Moist heat supplied by warm towels, hot packs, a bath or a shower can be used at home for 15 to 20 minutes three times a day to relieve symptoms.

◆ Cold supplied by a bag of ice or frozen vegetables wrapped in a towel helps to stop pain and reduce swelling when used for 10 to 15 minutes at a time.

◆ Hydrotherapy (water therapy) can decrease pain and stiffness. Exercising in a large pool may be easier because water takes some weight off painful joints.

◆ Mobilization therapies include traction (gentle, steady pulling), massage and manipulation (using the hands to restore normal movement to stiff joints).

◆ Relaxation therapy also helps reduce pain. Patients can learn to release the tension in their muscles to relieve pain.

◆ Acupuncture is a traditional Chinese method of pain relief in which a medically qualified acupuncturist places needles in certain sites. Researchers believe that the needles stimulate deep sensory nerves that tell the brain to release natural painkillers (endorphins).

How often should people with arthritis exercise?

◆ Range-of-motion exercises can be done daily and should be done at least every other day.

◆ Strengthening exercises should be done every other day unless you have severe pain or swelling in your joints.

◆ Endurance exercises should be done for 20 to 30 minutes three times a week unless you have severe pain or swelling in your joints.

How much exercise is too much?

Most experts agree that if exercise causes pain that lasts for more than one hour, then it is too strenuous. People with arthritis should work with their physiotherapist or doctor to adjust their exercise programme if they notice any:

◆ unusual or persistent fatigue

◆ increased weakness

◆ decreased range of motion

◆ continuing pain (pain that lasts more than two hours after exercising).

What could happen if I don't exercise?

If your joints hurt, you may not feel like exercising. However, if you don't exercise, your joints can become even more stiff and painful. Exercise is beneficial because it keeps your muscles, bones and joints healthy.

Because you have osteoarthritis, it is important to keep your muscles as strong as possible. The stronger the muscles and tissue are around your joints, the better they will be able to support and protect those joints – even those that are weak and damaged from osteoarthritis. If you don't exercise, your muscles become smaller and weaker.

Many people with osteoarthritis keep painful joints in a bent position because at first it's more comfortable, but if your joints stay in one position for too long (without movement), you may lose your ability to straighten them. Exercise helps keep your joints flexible, allowing you to continue to do your daily tasks as independently as possible.

Exercise can change your mood. If you're in pain, you may feel depressed. If you feel depressed, you may not feel like moving or exercising – but without exercise, you may feel more pain and depression. Research has shown that participating in a regular exercise programme is a great way to feel better and move more comfortably.

Two particular forms of exercise that have proved beneficial to people with osteoarthritis are yoga and t'ai chi. These can involve range-of-motion and strengthening exercises and can become a type of lifestyle activity, which can be done anywhere for any period of time that is appropriate.

Yoga

Yoga is a set of theories and practices with origins in ancient India. Literally, the word yoga comes from a Sanskrit word meaning 'to yoke' or 'to unite'. It focuses on unifying the mind, body and spirit, and fostering greater self-awareness and connection between the individual and their surroundings.

As interest in yoga has increased in Western countries over the last few decades, yoga postures are increasingly practised solely for physical health benefits. This physical practice of yoga, often called hatha yoga, sometimes overlaps or includes references to the other aspects of yoga, such as meditative practices. A popular misconception is that yoga focuses merely on increasing flexibility. The practice of hatha yoga also emphasizes postural alignment, strength, endurance and balance.

Today's yoga participants are young and old, flexible and inflexible, shapely and out of shape – everyday people who want to treat their bodies and minds well. Numerous scientific trials on yoga have been published in major medical journals. These studies have shown that yoga is a safe and effective way to increase physical activity and also has important psychological benefits due to its meditative nature. As with other forms of exercise, yoga can increase muscle strength, improve flexibility, enhance respiratory endurance and promote balance. Yoga is also associated with increased energy and fewer bodily aches and pains. Finally, yoga is associated with increased mental energy as well as positive feelings (such as alertness and enthusiasm), and fewer negative feelings (reduced excitability, anxiety, aggressiveness) and somatic complaints. In summary, yoga is associated with a wide range of physical and psychological benefits that may be especially helpful for persons living with osteoarthritis. Yoga poses can help strengthen your joints and the muscles around them, which is crucial in preventing and dealing with osteoarthritis. It also increases the range of motion in joints thus reducing the risk of stiffness.

A core concept of yoga is that it is not competitive or goal-oriented; it is about tuning into your own body and its limitations and doing what it needs on a particular day. Ideally your yoga teacher (assuming you are in a class) will emphasize the importance of approaching your yoga practice with this awareness.

While there are some yoga poses that do require a great deal of flexibility, strength and balance, those poses should only be attempted by very experienced yogis and are not for beginners or people with physical limitations.

Again, a good yoga teacher will provide alternatives and modifications to all activities so that students can work within their levels of comfort.

The general rule for people with osteoarthritis is that if it hurts, stop. The old adage of 'no pain, no gain' does not apply to yoga, particularly if you have physical limitations. When doing backbends, people with back pain should keep them relatively small. For those with arthritis of the hip, be cautious when doing 'hip openers' or poses with extreme external rotation of the hips. Generally, you will notice pain if you are going too far with the pose, but sometimes the effects are not felt until the next day. It is important to be gentle with your practice, especially at first. If you do not experience any pain after a few days, you can decide to gradually increase the intensity of the poses. As with any condition, it is important to be cautious and pay attention to your body and consult your doctor before commencing the programme. Also, be sure to consult your doctor and instructor if you experience any pain or difficulty resulting from yoga practice.

T'ai chi

T'ai chi is an ancient Chinese practice designed to exercise the body, mind and spirit. Moving through t'ai chi positions gently works muscles, focuses concentration and, according to Chinese philosophy, improves the flow of '*qi*', the vital life energy that sustains health and calms the mind (*qi* is pronounced 'chee' and is often spelled 'chi'). Chinese medicine is based on the belief that disease is due to blocks or imbalances in the flow of *qi*.

Chinese medicine incorporates the use of acupuncture, herbs and t'ai chi in the belief they can help balance the flow of *qi*, and, in doing so, cure illness and maintain health.

In the thirteenth century, Taoist priest Chang San Fang observed a crane fighting with a snake and compared their movements to yin and yang. Some t'ai chi movements are said to mimic those of the animals. In China, where ta'i chi has been practised for some 600 years, t'ai chi isn't just a feel-good workout but a therapy, preventive measure and remedy for almost every ailment, including osteoarthritis. Given its low impact and evidence that it tends to increase muscle strength and balance and give general pain relief, t'ai chi is a worthwhile option for many people with osteoarthritis.

Along with other Chinese imports, such as acupuncture and herbs, t'ai chi is becoming popular in the West. It appeals to people of all ages because it's not intimidating. Seniors particularly like t'ai chi because the slow, synchronized movements are easy to learn and to perform.

T'ai chi movements are based on shifting body weight through a series of light, controlled movements that flow rhythmically together into one long, graceful gesture. The sequences have poetic names, such as 'waving hand in the cloud' or 'pushing the mountain', and can be quite beautiful to an observer. T'ai chi takes the joints through their range of motion gently, while the emphasis on breathing and inner stillness relieves stress and anxiety.

Classes are inexpensive, and it can be practised almost anywhere at any time, with no special equipment or clothing.

T'ai chi classes are usually small, with fewer than 20 people of diverse ages. It's common to see people in their 80s alongside students in their 20s and every age in between.

There are five distinct styles of t'ai chi and many variations within each style. The most gentle and, therefore, most suitable styles for people with osteo-arthritis, are the Yang, Sun, Wu and Hao styles. Beginners should avoid the Chen style, which is more brisk and active and not recommended for most people with arthritis.

You may encounter a t'ai chi class that teaches a variation on a style or one that combines several styles. The 'right' version for you is one that you can do easily, without making hard or forceful movements and without stressing your joints or muscles.

T'ai chi classes usually last about one hour, and may be held once or twice a week. They begin with a gentle warm-up and breathing exercises or a medita-tion to quiet the mind.

The teacher demonstrates individual poses and then leads the class through the sequences, step by step, gradually linking the movements together in longer sequences. The sequences can be done slowly, or with more speed and energy, but movements are always soft and graceful, with careful attention to breath-ing and posture. The movements are inspired by the martial arts, but require no jumping or jerking of the body.

Classes end with cooling-down exercises and, sometimes, a short meditation. At the end of class, you should feel relaxed. If you have pain that lasts more than a few hours after class, talk to the instructor about how to change the movements to work within your limits.

T'ai chi has been shown to decrease pain and joint stiffness, and improve physical function and balance in people with osteoarthritis (Song *et al.* 2003). The 'Sun-style' t'ai chi reported on in this study was designed specifically for patients with osteoarthritis. It involves slow, continuous, and gentle motions with a higher stance than other t'ai chi styles.

Sore muscles, sprains and electrical sensations have been reported rarely with t'ai chi. T'ai chi should not be used as a substitute for more proven therapies for potentially severe medical conditions. Consult a qualified health care provider if you experience dizziness, shortness of breath, chest pain, headache or severe pain related to t'ai chi.

References

Bartels, E. M. (2006) Aquatic exercise for the treatment of knee and hip osteoarthritis. *Cochrane Database of Systematic Reviews* 4.

Brosseau, L. (2006) Intensity of exercise for the treatment of osteoarthritis. *Cochrane Database of Systematic Reviews* 4.

Song, R., Lee, E. O., Lam, P., Bae, S. C., Song, R., Lee, E. O. *et al.* (2003) Effects of t'ai chi exercise on pain, balance, muscle strength, and perceived difficulties in physical functioning in older women with osteoarthritis: a randomized clinical trial. *Journal of Rheumatology* 30(9): 2039–44.

10

Diet

For many years researchers have been exploring the link between diet and osteoarthritis. We continue to hear claims that special diets, foods and supplements may help to cure or alleviate symptoms of osteoarthritis, but most claims are unproven. Many experts speculate that claims of nutritional remedies and cures with food or dietary supplements are related to the 'placebo effect', which is when the patient *perceives* that their symptoms and well-being have improved after new therapy, regardless of evidence for actual physical improvement.

Because there is little scientific evidence confirming the benefits of modified diets for patients with osteoarthritis, health professionals are cautious about recommending these types of dietary manipulations to their patients.

However, there are others with limited or no medical background who will provide advice about the benefits of diets for osteoarthritis. The advice given is often questionable, expensive and can be dangerous.

In short, there is a lot of confusing advice in magazines and books on diet and many food supplements that reportedly help with osteoarthritis. Some people end up taking expensive food supplements or eat elaborate diets that do not help, or may even be harmful. Often the best results can be achieved by simpler, cheaper methods. If you have osteoarthritis the most important guidelines on diet are that you attain a balanced diet, include foods that contain essential fatty acids (one aspect of the diet that can have a beneficial effect), and keep your weight at a healthy level. In addition, many with OA are overweight or obese and caloric restriction is a vital ingredient of any weight-loss programme. The information you need to follow these guidelines is included below, as well as some background facts that dispel some commonly held misconceptions.

A balanced diet

The right diet can certainly help some people with OA. Until we have access to more conclusive data regarding the benefits of dietary manipulation for OA, patients are encouraged to follow a healthy, balanced diet that fosters a healthy weight. The main messages are as follows:

◆ Eat a variety of foods.

◆ Balance the food you eat with physical activity to maintain or improve your weight.

◆ Choose a diet with plenty of grain products, vegetables and fruits.

◆ Choose a diet low in fat, particularly saturated fat and cholesterol.

◆ Choose a diet moderate in sugars.

◆ Ensure you are getting adequate omega-3 fatty acids, and vitamins D and K in your diet.

NOTE: Avoid elimination diets and faddy nutritional practices and be cautious of claims of miracle cures.

Weight control

The most important single link between your diet and OA is certainly your weight. Being overweight puts an extra burden on the weight-bearing joints (the back, hips, knees, ankles and feet) when they are already damaged or under strain. Because of the way joints work, the effect of the weight can be four or five times greater in important parts of the joint. For example, being only 4.5 kilograms overweight increases the force on the knee by 13– 27 kilograms with each step. If you are overweight and have OA in any of your

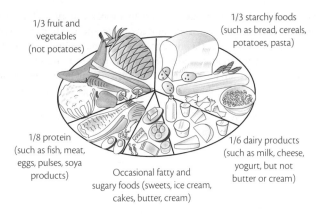

1/3 fruit and vegetables (not potatoes)

1/3 starchy foods (such as bread, cereals, potatoes, pasta)

1/8 protein (such as fish, meat, eggs, pulses, soya products)

Occasional fatty and sugary foods (sweets, ice cream, cakes, butter, cream)

1/6 dairy products (such as milk, cheese, yogurt, but not butter or cream)

Figure 10.1 Eat a diet that has the right balance of different types of food. Proportions are by weight. Source: http://www.arc.org.uk/arthinfo/patpubs/6010/6010.asp

weight-bearing joints, losing weight will help you more than any food supplements. The combination of weight loss and exercise has been shown in clinical trials to provide large improvements in knee OA symptoms (pain and mobility).

Being overweight is a clear risk factor for developing OA, and the increasing and worsening of symptoms of existing disease. Overweight women have nearly four times the risk of knee OA; for overweight men the risk is five times greater.

How do I know if I am overweight?

The use of the body mass index (BMI) as an indicator of healthy and unhealthy weights is based on extensive research linking the index with associated health risks. Your BMI is calculated by dividing your weight in kilograms by the square of your height in metres. According to the new guidelines from the National Institute of Health (NIH), someone with a BMI of 25–29.9 is overweight, while obesity is a BMI of greater than 30. (A BMI of 30 is about 15 kg overweight). You should aim for a BMI of less than 25.

What is the best way to lose weight?

Slimming has become big business. There are many slimming treatments and so-called miracle diets, and this can be confusing. Unfortunately there is no miracle cure. Crash and fad diets are usually unbalanced and are not recommended. Most people find they put weight back on when they return to normal eating. *The only way to lose weight permanently is to change what you eat.*

To work normally, your body needs food to supply energy and a variety of vitamins and minerals. If your diet contains more energy than you burn up, your body will convert the extra energy to fat and you will put on weight. On the other hand, if your food contains less energy than you are using, you will lose weight. If you are unable to take as much exercise as before because of your OA or other health problems, you need less energy and should eat less.

The energy in food is measured in kilocalories (kcal)—sometimes just called calories. If you eat fewer calories, it is important not to eat less vitamins and minerals at the same time. This is why it is important to eat foods that have a lot of vitamins and minerals per calorie, such as fruit and vegetables.

Cut down on the fat you eat

Fat has twice as many calories as the same weight of starch or protein.

Most people eat far more fat than they need for health. Eating one ounce (about 30 grams) less fat each day saves 252 calories! So cutting calories does not require massive sacrifices. Making minor changes in the foods you eat can do the trick.

The fats in food are of three kinds: saturates, monounsaturates and polyunsaturates. Saturates are found mostly in biscuits, cheese, cooking fats, hard margarine, pastry, pies, meat fat, full-fat milk, dairy products and chips. Some vegetable fats are also mainly saturates. Saturated fats are the most important kind of fat to reduce: the body doesn't need them and they may actually aggravate OA. Softer fats and oils have more monosaturates and polyunsaturates but just as many calories, so limiting them is still important to lose weight.

To eat less fat, follow these rules:

◆ Look out for and avoid 'invisible' fats in foods such as biscuits, cakes, chocolate, pastry and savoury snacks—check the labels.

◆ Trim fat off any meat you eat.

◆ Always choose lean cuts of meat.

◆ Choose fish and poultry more often.

◆ Use low-fat milk (skimmed or semi-skimmed).

◆ Use low-fat spreads.

◆ Grill instead of frying foods.

◆ Fill up on cereals, fruit and vegetables.

Cut down on sugar

Sugar contains only calories and has no other food value (so-called empty calories) so it can be cut down without any loss of nourishment. Eating one ounce (about 30 grams) less sugar each day saves 112 calories! Try not to add sugar to drinks and cereals. Although artificial sweeteners contain very few calories, it is better to get used to food being less sweet by not adding them to drinks. Dried fruit like raisins can be used to sweeten cereals and puddings: unlike sugar and artificial sweeteners, they also provide vitamins and minerals.

Eat more fruit and vegetables

The World Health Organisation recommends that we should have at least five portions of fruit and vegetables every day. This is to make sure that the body receives the important antioxidants and vitamins which it needs to protect it during the stress of disease. Eating plenty of fruit and vegetables, especially the brightly coloured varieties like carrots, tomatoes, beetroot and broccoli, also provides you with more fibre. Remember, you also get fibre from wholegrain versions of bread, cereals, pasta and rice. These foods are more filling so they will also help if you are trying to lose weight!

Take regular exercise

Exercise is very important. Not only does it involve you using up calories which would otherwise end up as fat, but it increases your strength and suppleness. Exercise is good for your general health, especially the heart and circulation. Of course, OA can make exercise difficult and painful, and the wrong kind of exercise can make it worse. But exercise does *not* have to mean running a marathon! A daily walk for half an hour with the dog or a walk to the local shops or park is exercise and it will help.

Many people find particular types of exercise suit them best. Some prefer swimming because being in water takes the weight off the joints; others prefer keep-fit classes, yoga or cycling. The most important thing is that you enjoy it and do it *regularly*. (See Chapter 9)

What about weight-loss medications?

Clinical guidelines suggest that all patients try lifestyle-based (diet and exercise) approaches for weight loss for at least six months before embarking on drug therapy.

Weight-loss drugs for long-term use may be tried as part of a comprehensive weight-loss programme that includes dietary therapy and physical activity in carefully selected patients (BMI greater than 30 without additional risk factors, BMI greater than 27 with two or more risk factors) who have been unable to lose weight or maintain weight loss with conventional non-drug therapies. In general, if a patient does not lose 2 kilograms in the first four weeks of treatment, the patient can be considered a non-responder to pharmacotherapy. Drug therapy may also be used during the weight-maintenance phase of treatment. Safety and effectiveness beyond one year of total treatment have not been established. Surgical management is yet another option that typically is reserved for the morbidly obese.

Essential fatty acids

One of the most exciting recent discoveries is that certain kinds of oil in the diet help some people with OA. These oils contain essential fatty acids (EFAs). Essential means that the body cannot make them for itself and must get them from food. The body uses these EFAs to make chemicals called prostaglandins and leukotrienes, the right balance of which has been shown to decrease cartilage loss, decrease the activity of enzymes that breakdown cartilage and decrease the expression of mediators of inflammation (inflammatory molecules). All of these factors may explain the beneficial effects of omega 3 in OA.

There are two groups of EFAs: omega 3, found mostly in fish oil; and omega 6, found mostly in plant seed oils. The typical Western diet is rich in omega 6 but does not contain enough omega 3.

Omega 3 EFAs are found naturally in oily fish, especially mackerel, sardines, pilchards and salmon, so it is a good idea to eat oily fish (for some the smell may be troublesome) three or four times a week. They can also be found in flaxseeds and flaxseed oil, walnuts and canola oil. The main omega-3 EFAs are called EPA and DHA, and most chemists and health food shops sell fish-oil capsules which contain high concentrations of these. Fish liver oil (cod or halibut) also contains these EFAs as well as vitamin D, which helps the body to absorb calcium.

But fish liver oils also contain a lot of vitamin A. This is dangerous in large amounts, and in particular should not be taken by pregnant women, or women who might become pregnant, because vitamin A can harm the unborn baby. Women in these groups should not take fish liver oils or vitamin A supplements at all. In most of the studies using fish oils, benefits are not usually observed until at least 12 weeks of continuous use and appear to increase with extended treatment time.

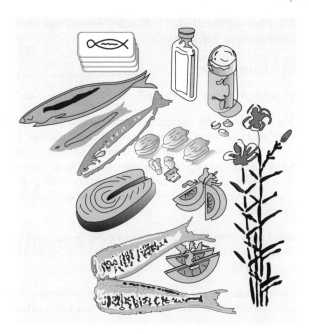

Figure 10.2 Oily fish and some plant seed oils are sources of omega-3 polyunsaturated fatty acids. Source: http://www.arc.org.uk/arthinfo/patpubs/6010/6010.asp

The main omega-6 EFA is called GLA. The best-known source is evening primrose oil, but several other plant seed oils also contain it (safflower, sunflower and corn oil). Again these are available from most chemists and health-food shops, but as we have already suggested, your diet probably contains enough omega 6 and you will only need to supplement omega 3.

Are there side-effects of EFAs?

In theory, EFAs can cause a problem by generating chemicals that cause free radicals in the body, which could lead to heart and circulation disease. Antioxidants are a group of vitamins and minerals that protect the body from this. They are found mostly in fresh fruit and vegetables, especially the brightly coloured varieties like carrots, tomatoes, beetroot and broccoli. Most chemists and health food shops stock antioxidant vitamin and mineral supplements.

It is also important to note that fish-oil supplements may interfere with blood clotting and increase the risk for stroke, especially when consumed in conjunction with aspirin or other non-steroidal anti-inflammatory drugs.

Taking fish oils has also been linked to changes in bowel habits such as diarrhoea, and may cause an upset stomach.

Other micronutrients

It is also important to ensure your diet has sufficient vitamin D and K.

Vitamin D is responsible for normal bone metabolism and potentially has effects on cartilage metabolism. In some studies an intake less than 258 IU/day (low intake) has been associated an increased risk of progression, blood levels less than 30 ng/ml (low level) have been associated with an increased risk of progression, osteophyte growth and cartilage loss, and associated with pain and decreased physical function. Furthermore improving blood levels of vitamin D improves physical function.

Recommended daily vitamin D requirements differ by age such that adults aged 19–50 years are recommended to get 200 IU/day, adults 51–70 years 400 IU/day, and adults 71 years and older 600 IU/day.

Vitamin D is synthesized in the skin under the action of sunlight. You can also get it in certain foods: in particular milk is often fortified with vitamin D.

Some common causes of vitamin D deficiency include:

- dark skin
- ageing
- wearing too much sunscreen, covering all exposed skin (some religions recommend particular dress-codes like this) and not getting outside (such as institutionalized people living in nursing homes)
- obesity (this is a fat-soluble (dissolves in fat) vitamin the more fat you have the more you need).

Vitamin K is responsible for normal bone metabolism and potentially has effects on cartilage metabolism. In some studies low blood levels of vitamin K have been associated with an increased prevalence of knee and hand osteoarthritis. The recommended vitamin K requirements are males 120 μg/day and females 90 μg/day. Some dietary sources that are rich in vitamin K include soybeans, spinach, blueberries and kale.

Common misconceptions about diet and arthritis

❓ Questions and answers

Q 1.   Should I take extra calcium if I have arthritis?

A.   Calcium is an important basic nutrient and not enough of it in the diet contributes to osteoporosis (brittle bones). Women after the menopause are particularly liable to osteoporosis. People with OA are statistically at lower risk of developing osteoporosis. If you are at risk the richest source of calcium in most people's diet is milk and dairy products (foods made from milk: cheese, yoghurt, etc., but *not* butter). If you have about 600 ml of milk per day or use other dairy products regularly, you should be getting enough calcium. Remember that skimmed milk contains more calcium than full-fat milk. A daily intake of calcium of 1000 mg or 1500 mg if you are over 60 is recommended. The table below can guide you on how much calcium is contained in some of the common dietary foods.

Calcium content of common foods*

◆ 0.2 litre (1/3 pint) whole milk 220 mg

◆ 0.2 litre (1/3 pint) semi-skimmed milk 230 mg

◆ 30 g (1 oz) hard cheese 190 mg

◆ 150 g (5 oz) carton low-fat yoghurt 225 mg

◆ 60 g (2 oz) sardines (including the bones) 310 mg

◆ 3 large slices brown or white bread 100 mg

◆ 3 large slices wholemeal bread 55 mg

◆ 115 g (4 oz) cottage cheese 80 mg

◆ 115 g (4 oz) baked beans 60 mg

◆ 115 g (4 oz) boiled cabbage 40 mg

* Figures provided are estimates only.

If, for any reason, you do not take many dairy products, soya milk is now available in most supermarkets and can be used in exactly the same way as cows' milk. Some soya milk is fortified with calcium, and these are the better ones to have. If you are not taking dairy products or a good quantity of soya milk, you may need a calcium supplement. Discuss this with a dietitian or your doctor.

Q 2. Should I take iron tablets if I have arthritis?

A. Iron is important to prevent anaemia. Many people with OA are anaemic, but this will not always be helped by iron tablets. The anaemia can be due to different causes. NSAIDs (non-steroidal anti-inflammatory drugs) such as aspirin, ibuprofen and diclofenac help pain related to OA but may cause stomach ulcers and bleeding in some people, leading to anaemia. If you are anaemic your doctor will advise you if you need more iron.

The best source of iron in food is red meat. However, as many people are now cutting down on red meat for various reasons, it is important to have iron from other sources. Iron from fish is easily absorbed by your body and oily fish are a very good source. For example, sardines contain as much iron as beef! Iron is better absorbed if there is also vitamin C in the meal so have a good portion of vegetables or salad or fresh fruit with your meal. On the other hand, tea reduces the amount of iron that your body can absorb so it is a good idea not to drink tea with your meal. If you are vegetarian, remember that dairy products like milk and cheese are a very poor source of iron, but pulses like haricot beans and lentils and dark leafy vegetables (such as spinach and watercress) are quite a good source. They should be included daily in a vegetarian diet.

Q3. Is it true that certain foods can make arthritis worse?

A. The best evidence we have that food can influence arthritis is from people with gout. Gout is a particular type of arthritis where the body is not able to properly absorb those foods that contain purines. This results in too much uric acid, which can crystallize in the joints. Drugs have largely replaced diet as a treatment for gout, but, if you have this condition, you can avoid the main sources of purines in the diet—do not eat liver, heart, kidney, meat extract, anchovies, crab, fish roe, herring, mackerel, sardines, shrimps and whitebait.

Alcohol particularly affects uric acid and people with gout should drink no alcohol at all or very little.

There has been some recent research about the effect of leaving certain foods out of the diet in other forms of arthritis. Fasting by eliminating certain foods from the diet is a very high-risk, short-term treatment and is currently not an accepted approach for the treatment of OA.

11

Glucosamine, vitamins, and osteoarthritis

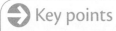 Key points

- Glucosamine sulphate, chondroitin sulphate and some vitamins are widely used in the field of osteoarthritis.

- There is evidence that they may reduce pain when taken for prolonged periods.

- They are well tolerated in most patients.

- More research is required before routinely recommending their use in all patients.

- It is the responsibility of each person to understand the mechanism, dose and potential side-effects behind each preparation before deciding if it is a treatment they wish to follow.

Today in both Europe and America, there are vast numbers of health food shops and mail order companies promoting herbal supplements and vitamins which they claim can improve our general well-being and also help specific conditions such as osteoarthritis. Doctors and nurses are frequently asked 'Will supplements help with my osteoarthritis?', and although there has been extensive research with their use in some diseases, to date research in the field of osteoarthritis is lagging behind. All conventional medicines go through extensive research and vigorous regulatory controls before being licensed and are closely monitored with regard to their efficacy and safety profile after being licensed for use in patients. This enables doctors to review the literature and establish the overall health benefits of each drug. Supplements, however, do not have to abide by such rigorous controls, making it difficult for doctors to give advice regarding many of the supplements that are available today.

The aim of this chapter is to provide information regarding the most frequently used supplements available today for osteoarthritis with the research that we have available. It is thought that there are three main areas where supplements can play a role in either improving symptoms or preventing further progression of osteoarthritis:

1. Preventing oxidative damage.

2. Preventing or repairing damaged cartilage.

3. Reducing inflammation.

An oxidant is an oxidizing agent that can potentially be damaging to its surrounding structures. In the joints oxidants are produced by the chondrocytes (cells in the cartilage): they target the main structure in the connective tissue of the joint (collagen) and depolarize the lubricant (the hyaluronate fliud) in the joint. Oxidants are therefore unwanted visitors to the joint.

Glucosamine and chondroitin

These are the two leading supplements in the field of osteoarthritis today, and rank third in the top-selling nutritional supplements in the USA. It is thought that one or another of these products is used by 5–8 per cent of American adults. In most of Europe they are available only with prescription, however in the USA and the UK they can be obtained via health food shops, in supermarkets and via home catalogue shopping companies. They can be found in a combined formulation or be bought separately. As with many medications, supplements and treatments they may not be beneficial for everyone, and it is necessary to have a trial period of about three months if they are to be taken for pain relief.

Glucosamine

There are two types of glucosamine available:

1. Glucosamine sulphate.

2. Glucosamine hydrochloride (a formulation suitable for vegetarians).

Glucosamine sulphate naturally occurs in the body, but the commercially available preparations are derived from shell fish such as crab, lobster and shrimp shells: if you have an allergy to shellfish it should be avoided, and vegetarians may choose glucosamine hydrochloride as an alternative. The recommended daily dose of glucosamine sulphate is 1500 mg per day: patients should be aware that over the counter medicataions vary the dose strength of each tablet. Patients who take glucosamine sulphate generally find the pain relief takes longer to achieve than regular non-steroidal anti-inflammatory drugs, varying between two weeks and three months, with the latter probably the most common duration. The pain-relieving effects can also last for up to three months after stopping it.

Most of the research conducted has used glucosamine sulphate and has tended to focus on patients with osteoarthritis of the knee. Although not all studies have shown benefit in pain relief over and above a dummy tablet (a placebo), the majority do show it to be effective in reducing pain over prolonged periods of time with pain relief consistent with mild anti-inflammatory medication. There is also emerging evidence that it may reduce the loss of cartilage in patients with knee OA and eventually reduce the need for knee replacement surgery if taken long term. There is less research on glucosamine hydrochloride, however early results from a large US study failed to demonstrate any significant benefit.

It is thought that glucosamine sulphate is a safe supplement to take but there are a couple of groups who should be careful if considering it:

◆ Those allergic to shellfish would be advised to avoid it due to a possible allergic reaction.

◆ It should be avoided in pregnancy or if breastfeeding due to a lack of research regarding its safety for the baby and mother.

There have been some concerns in the past that glucosamine may raise blood sugar levels in those who have diabetes, although studies to date have dispelled this. However it is wise to closely monitor blood sugar levels whilst taking glucosamine if you have diabetes and to avoid its use in patients with unstable diabetes.

Chondroitin

Chondroitin sulphate, like glucosamine sulphate, is a naturally occurring substance found in the body and is a part of a protein that gives cartilage its elasticity. The preparations for sale commercially can be derived from one of three sources:

◆ avian

◆ bovine

◆ shark.

It is thought to have similar effects to that of glucosamine sulphate in that it can reduce the pain levels and also play a role in the formation and repair of cartilage in mild to moderate osteoarthritis. A number of studies have been performed, and although they do not universally demonstrate significant pain relief over and above placebo, overall it appears to induce pain relief to a similar degree as glucosamine sulphate. Again there is early evidence that it may prevent further cartilage loss and hence prevent disease progression in patients with knee osteoarthritis.

It too has a good safety record, although like glucosamine it should not be used in pregnancy or if breastfeeding, as no studies have been conducted with these groups of people. It is suggested that those people who take blood-thinning agents, such as heparin, warfarin or aspirin, should have their clotting time monitored. Chondroitin has a similar structure to heparin and so could cause bleeding in some people. The recommended dose to take is 800 mg per day.

Vitamins

Some vitamins are antioxidants whose role it is to suppress the oxidants present in the joint from causing joint damage and thereby help to relieve the symptoms of osteoarthritis. Most vitamins are to be found in a well-balanced diet and in fact are absorbed better by ingesting them in this way as opposed to taking supplements. The three main vitamins thought to be involved in relieving osteoarthritis are vitamins C, D and E.

Vitamin C

Vitamin C is an antioxidant and therefore counteracts the oxidants that damage the cartilage. It has also been shown to play a role in the production of the collagen that is present in cartilage, and this has been supported by a study that revealed those with a low level of vitamin C had a poorer quality of cartilage. Vitamin C is present in fruit and vegetables and it is recommended that we all have five portions of these a day.

Vitamin E

It is thought that vitamin E acts in an anti-inflammatory role in the osteoarthritic joint and therefore may be effective in reducing pain, although the data is conflicting regarding its benefit.

Vitamin D

Vitamin D has an extensive role to play in the bones and joints: most research has been conducted in the field of osteoporosis where its benefits are substantial.

Early research has suggested that vitamin D may also be important in osteoarthritis, where it is thought to have a role to play in the disease progression. Vitamin D affects most components of the joint including bone, cartilage and muscle, and may therefore have multiple effects on its structure and function. Research has found that those subjects with a low dietary intake of vitamin D, or low levels in the body, have an accelerated progression of the disease. The majority of vitamin D is produced in the skin in response to exposure to sunlight, although it is also absorbed from food. With the increasing, and appropriate, adoption of sun-avoidance behaviour, the rates of vitamin D deficiency, especially in the elderly, are substantial and rising. Most societies recommend that a supplement of 400 IU of vitamin D per day is a safe amount to take.

Other supplements

There have been small studies on a number of less common supplements and their effects on osteoarthritis, some of which have been positive, but more research is necessary. These supplements include the avocado and soya bean, S-adenosylmethionine (SAM-e), and ginger.

Conclusion

Many of the nutritional supplements available today claim to have benefits for those with osteoarthritis, but it is important to remember that the research in this field can be scanty and poorly conducted compared to the vigorous field of conventional medicines. Dietitians would agree that most vitamins can be acquired through a healthy diet of fresh fruit and vegetables, fish oils and natural sunshine, and that overdosing could occur if unnecessary supplements are taken above the required diet.

Although some clinicians are not convinced of the benefits of glucosamine and chondroitin in relation to osteoarthritis, in general they have a high safety record and it is accepted that these two supplements can be considered for those with osteoarthritis. Each individual is responsible for what they choose to take and are advised to research their benefits before investing in this field. Medications used in other diseases should not be stopped without first discussing this with your doctor.

12

Medicines used in osteoarthritis

➡ Key points

◆ The medicines available today are predominantly used to treat the symptoms and not to cure osteoarthritis.

◆ These medicines should be used alongside the other strategies in the management of osteoarthritis.

◆ Although some medicines are beneficial in relieving the symptoms associated with osteoarthritis, they can carry unwanted side-effects.

◆ It is important to understand the role medications can play in the management of your osteoarthritis and to discuss this with your doctor.

There are many medicines used to help in the management of osteoarthritis, but sadly so far there is no 'magic tablet' that can cure the condition. The medications available are aimed at reducing the unpleasant symptoms that OA causes, such as stiffness and pain, and there is a vast array of medications on the market in this field. However, the general approach by doctors is that using medication in conjunction with other management strategies such as exercising and pacing is the most beneficial approach.

The aim of this chapter is to give an overview of the medicines most commonly used in OA and how they should be taken.

In what forms are medications available?

With advances in technology, there are many different ways that medications can be taken. In OA the most common mode is by mouth, in either tablet form or liquid, as this is the most convenient, cheapest and also the least invasive route (when compared to injections or suppositories). It also allows the person more control of the administration of the medicine. Some strong pain-relieving medicines come in patch form, and there are also some medicines used in OA that can be administered in the form of creams. Some treatments, such as corticosteroids, can be given by injection directly into the joint.

Medicines used outside their licence

All medicines that are available on prescription have gone through rigorous compulsory stages of research and development during which time the drug is registered for a specific licence for a specific use. However it is not uncommon for doctors to use drugs outside their licence in their practice if there is research to support it, for example amitryptyline (see below).

How to take the medication

Many people are not happy to take medication long term, either because they are concerned about side-effects, or because they are worried about becoming dependent on the drug, and many people simply do not like to take tablets. For these common reasons many people take their medication as and when they need it, and usually when the pain becomes severe. This often leads to peaks and troughs in pain levels, which results in having to take a higher dose of the painkillers in order to reduce the high levels of pain.

All tablets have a time limit as to how long they are effective for and this can vary from drug to drug: taking your medication on a regular basis will prevent the pain from spiralling out of control. Some people find in doing this that they can take smaller doses of the medication. By taking the medication on a regular basis you will hopefully find that you can take control the pain rather than the pain controlling you.

Pain-relieving medicines in general (analgesics)

There are many analgesics for pain in general on the market today and this alone can be quite baffling. Some are called by the generic name, some use the manufacturer's brand name, and some can contain more than one drug. In general there are three main groups of analgesia, which are categorized according to their strength. The easiest way to demonstrate this is to use a ladder model (see Fig. 12.1): the higher up the ladder, the stronger the analgesia.

The bottom rung of the ladder – non-opioid drugs

Generally speaking most people with osteoarthritis take medication from this group of drugs. However, it is important to know that although they are

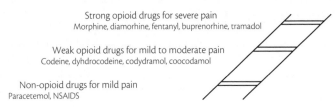

Figure 12.1 The analgesic ladder.

classed as medicines used for mild pain this does not mean they have mild side-effects. Taken in the correct dosage, paracetamol has few side-effects, however the non-steroidal anti-inflammatory drugs (NSAIDS) can have some serious unwanted side-effects, such that they are used sparingly in people who have osteoarthritis.

The middle rung of the ladder – weak opioid drugs

If the drugs designed for mild pain are unhelpful your doctor may suggest trying a drug from this group. As suggested by their title, these drugs are weak versions of opioids (opiods are derived from the poppy which produces opium). They are either manufactured on their own or combined with paracetamol. Unfortunately the side-effects of opioids can be unpleasant and can involve constipation, confusion, reduced cognitive function (slow thought processing) and hallucinations and insomnia, and hence are not always popular with patients.

The top rung of the ladder – strong opioid drugs

As their title suggests, these are the strongest opioids: they can be either synthetic or natural. Some drugs in this group are available in the form a patch worn by the patient, but most are available to take orally. These drugs have greater analgesic properties, but the unwanted side-effects can also be enhanced to such a degree that they outweigh any benefits. For some patients, especially the elderly, the side-effects could heighten the risk of falling.

With all opioids there are concerns about dependency, and for this reason only the very mild form of opioids are available over the counter: stronger opioids are prescribed by your doctor following a full assessment. People who take regular opioids should always be reviewed regularly by their prescribing doctor to monitor the effects, but it is equally important to seek clinical advice if you find that the dose of these strong opioids starts to escalate.

Starting your medication

Doctors will initially choose a mild form of analgesia to help with the pain and stiffness caused by osteoarthritis, and many people with this condition find that the drugs from the bottom rung of the ladder are adequate enough. However, if this fails to control the pain, either an increased dose or a stronger analgesia may be chosen using the ladder approach (Fig. 12.1).

There are many different types of analgesics in each group, and if one fails to help then the doctor may try another drug from that group. Unfortunately it is often the case that the higher up the ladder one goes the more severe and unpleasant the side-effects can be, and for many this can outweigh the benefits of taking the drug. It is therefore important to discuss the use of these drugs with your doctor.

Common medicines used in osteoarthritis

We will now look at the most common of these drugs used in the management of osteoarthritis.

Paracetamol/Acetaminophen

This is the recommended first-line drug of choice for mild to moderate pain caused by osteoarthritis. It is a safe drug to use so long as the maximum dose is not exceeded (1 g up to four times a day = 4 g in total). It is not an anti-inflammatory drug but is an analgesic. The side-effects are generally very mild but can include constipation for some people. There are some groups of people who should avoid using it, for instance those who have liver failure. Long term it is considered to be a safe drug to use, although some studies have found mild indigestion with a prolonged daily dose of 4 g. It is important to note that many flu remedies contain paracetamol and so it is important to read the small print to avoid overdosing.

Non-steroidal anti-inflammatory drugs (NSAIDS)

- Arthrotec

- Diclofenac

- Diflunisal

- Fenbrufen

- Ibuprofen

- Naproxen

- Piroxicam

- Indometacin

- Nabumetone

- Sulindac

- Ketorolac

- Meloxicam

- Ketoprofen

- Tenoxicam

- Aspirin.

Should Acetaminophen fail to help the pain in moderate to severe OA pain, NSAIDS are considered. These are anti-inflammatory drugs but they are not steroids (as the title suggests), they are also analgesics. It is thought they are effective in the management of osteoarthritis because of a combination of their analgesic and anti-inflammatory properties. They are effective in relieving osteoarthritic pain for many people, although long-term studies have shown paracetamol to be equally effective.

NSAIDs are considered to be a mild analgesic, however, this does not necessarily mean they have mild side-effects. In fact NSAIDS are a group of drugs that should be used with caution in the treatment of osteoarthritis due to the side-effects which include reduced kidney function, gastric tract (the stomach and small intestine) bleeding, and ulceration which could be fatal. More recently they have been shown to increase the chance of a myocardial infarction (heart attack) in prolonged use in patients who already have other risk factors for heart disease (see below).

The reason NSAIDS are associated with such side-effects is their mode of action. Prostaglandins are naturally produced in the body and are responsible for the inflammatory response to an injury or a disease, which is why NSAIDs are effective in relieving pain in these diseases. However, they also help to produce a natural protective lining for the gastric tract (the stomach and small intestine) from the body's own corrosive gastric acid that is produced to digest food. Prostaglandins are produced following a chain of events initiated by enzymes. The enzyme that initiates this action is called cyclooxygenase-1. NSAIDS block production of the prostaglandins by inhibiting this enzyme and although this stops the inflammatory response and eases pain, it also blocks the production of the gastric tract's protective fluid, causing heartburn and gastric discomfort and the side-effects mentioned previously. They are also influential in cardiovascular events as they can increase blood pressure and so cause hypertension, which can predispose a patient to heart attacks (myocardial infarctions).

There are some groups of people in whom NSAIDS should be used with extreme caution as the risk of side-effects can be increased:

- Those over 60 years.

- Those with a history of ulceration.

- Those on warfarin or blood-thinning agents.

- Those taking corticosteroids.

- Smokers.

- Those with a history of cardiovascular disease.

- Those with high blood pressure.

- Those who drink more than three units per day of alcohol.

- Those who are in general poor health.

There are several different groups of NSAIDS and within each group there are numerous tablets. There is not always any rhyme or reason as to why a particular NSAID will help one person but not suit another, and often the patient may have to try a few until the most beneficial one is found. However, it is very important not to administer more than one type of NSAID at any one time, as this would increase your risk of severe side-effects dramatically.

The advice given to people who take NSAIDS is to take the lowest possible dose for the shortest possible time and to take them with or after food. They should stop taking them immediately if gastric pain or upset occur. Some clinicians also co-prescribe a gastric protector with the NSAIDS to help protect the gastric tract, and some NSAIDS already come in a combined preparation with a gastric protector: for example, Arthrotec contains misopristol (a gastric protector). Some people find that NSAIDS can exacerbate their asthma and they should be avoided if this is the case.

NSAID creams

These have been found to be beneficial in hand or knee osteoarthritis but not so effective for hip osteoarthritis due to the inability for the cream to penetrate so deeply. Although there have been reports of serious gastric side-effects with NSAIDS, the cream has a good safety record. Unfortunately many people find that the benefits of the cream can wane, and it is thought it may play a role in managing pain during a flare-up as opposed to using it long term. Side-effects can include itching and rash but this usually disappears when use stops.

Selective Cox-2 medicines

- Celecoxib.

- Etoricoxib.

- Lumaricoxib.

These are also non-steroidal anti-inflammatory drugs, but unlike the NSAIDS discussed above they are less likely to cause gastric upset. The Cox-2 enzyme is responsible for inflammation but not for the production of gastric protection: inhibiting the Cox-2 enzyme can reduce inflammation but gastric protection is not altered. These are newer drugs than the NSAIDS and although they are safer than NSAIDS with regard to gastric side-effects, unfortunately they are no safer with regard to the cardiovascular system, and over recent years we have seen the withdrawal of Vioxx from long-term use for this reason.

As with traditional NSAIDs, this group of drugs can be very effective for people with osteoarthritis but it is important to weigh the risks of unwanted side-effects with the benefits. It is thought that they are relatively safe for short-term use but they are not desirable for long-term use, and there are groups of people in whom they should be used with extreme caution:

- Those with a history of heart disease or who have had a stroke.

- Those with a family history of heart disease.

- Those with hypertension.

- Those who smoke.

- Those with diabetes.

Amitriptyline

This is a common drug used in the management of chronic pain and it is particularly effective in treating sharp stabbing type pains that are caused by nerves. It was originally licensed for the treatment of depression when taken in high doses, however it was later found to have beneficial effects for reducing

115

pain when taken in lower doses (10–50 mg) and today is prescribed to many people with osteoarthritis alongside the analgesics mentioned in this chapter.

It is a drug that should be taken on a regular basis for it to be effective, as benefits are not always seen for a few days. It is often prescribed to be taken at night (2 hours before bedtime) as one of the side-effects is sleepiness: taking the drug in this way means the side-effect can be used to help have a good night's sleep! Some people develop a hung-over feeling for the first few days of starting it and clinicians often therefore advise people to take it in very small doses and gradually build up the dose until benefits are felt and side-effects minimal. During this period you need to ensure that you are safe to drive or operate machinery and your doctor will be able to give guidance on this.

The dose needed can vary from person to person, but the most common drug doses are between 10 and 50 mg each night. Side-effects can include a dry mouth and some people can develop water retention or weight gain. This drug is a prescription-only medication and there are some people for whom it is not recommended, for example those who have glaucoma or abnormal heart rhythms. Similarly there are some drugs with which it is contraindicated.

Capsaicin cream

This is derived from the seeds and membranes of the Nightshade family of plants, which includes the pepper plant, and it acts by desentisizing the C fibres (the nerves that carry the pain messages). It has been shown to be a safe medicine to use either in conjunction with the other analgesics or on its own. It can be prescribed in differing strengths and to achieve maximum benefit it should be applied 3–4 times a day.

Due to its origin it is common following the first application to experience pain, burning, redness and sometimes irritation to the area where the cream is applied, but this usually settles following further applications. Due to the nature of the side-effects it is recommended that hands are washed immediately following application and that the cream is kept away from the eye and not allowed in contact with broken skin. It is thought to have few side-effects other than the local skin reactions already mentioned and approximately 20 per cent of people who take it find it effective.

Conclusion

Many people find analgesics are very effective. Pain is a unique experience to each person and therefore the choice of analgesia that suits one person may not always be beneficial for everyone. It is important to note that many of the analgesics carry with them unwanted side-effects as well as benefits, and it is the responsibility of each individual, given the relevant information, to decide whether the benefits of taking the medication out weigh the side-effects.

We are all too often aware of new concerns and discoveries with some of the medications and the long-term side-effects that they can have and in recent years we have seen media reports and the withdrawal of some medications. Research and monitoring of drugs is always ongoing for our own safety and is the nature of progressive medicine. It is hoped that in future years scientists may be able to improve the safety of the drugs that many people find beneficial.

13

Injection therapies

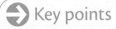 Key points

- Injections can lead to substantial reductions in pain.

- They should be administered by a trained practitioner.

- They should be used alongside other strategies for managing pain.

- Injections do not provide a cure for osteoarthritis.

Injections are used to help in the management of osteoarthritis, but they are not a cure for the condition. They act by reducing symptoms such as pain and discomfort with the aim of improving function once more. As with other medicines, they should be used as part of a package, for example alongside exercising, losing weight (if overweight) and pacing.

The injections that we will cover in this chapter are called intra-articular injections – injections directly into the joint itself. They are therefore very different to the usual intramuscular injections (e.g. the flu jab) or subcutaneous injections (e.g. those used to administer insulin). There are two intra-articular injections commonly used in the management of osteoarthritis:

- Corticosteroid injections.

- Hyaluronic acid.

This chapter will cover these two injections and look at how effective they are, who they are suitable for and potential side-effects.

Corticosteroid intra-articular injections

Corticosteroids are hormones that are either produced naturally by the adrenal gland (found above the kidney) or produced synthetically. Most injection preparations are synthetic. They have various metabolic functions, but are used in osteoarthritis because of their potent ability to reduce inflammation.

They were first used in the 1950s and to date most studies have concentrated on the knee joint, although there are some indications that it may also be beneficial for hips. The vast majority of the research conducted with the knee joint confirms that corticosteroid injections are beneficial when compared to a placebo treatment. Today approximately 53 per cent of doctors use these injections to help alleviate the pain caused by osteoarthritis.

Who are they suitable for?

It is thought that corticosteroid injections are most beneficial in those people who are having a flare-up of pain and/or who have an effusion (sewlling) of the knee. The EULAR (European) guidelines recommend that these injections should be used for people with a flare-up of knee pain who fail to respond to conventional NSAIDS or other analgesia. There are some people for whom the injection would not be suitable, for example those with bleeding disorders, those taking anticoagulants and those who have a skin infection.

How effective are they and how often can they be given?

As mentioned earlier, the corticosteroid injection is not a cure for osteoarthritis but it can help relieve the pain and inflammation. The onset of pain reduction is usually rapid (between 24–48 hours) with the maximum effect being reached within a few days. Studies have shown that the benefits last up to four weeks in most subjects and up to three months in some patients who have effusions of the knee. They can be repeated up to four times per year for the knee joint although usually less often for hand joints. Research to date has not shown repeated injections to cause any deterioration of the osteoarthritis in humans. However, animal studies have shown that corticosteroids speeds up the progression of the underlying structural changes associated with OA.

Safety

It is the responsibility of the doctor to discuss any potential complications prior to any procedure. As with any injection into a joint, there is always a risk that infection could be introduced which can cause septic arthritis. The risk of this is thought to be relatively low (1: 14,000), but is a risk nonetheless which can result in increased symptoms and rarely death. It is important therefore that the injections are performed by a proficient and qualified doctor who is aware of the sterile technique required.

Side-effects

It is not uncommon following the injection to have a temporary, mild flare-up of knee pain occasionally accompanied by some inflammation. This is due to a natural reaction of the synovial fluid in the joint to the crystal steroid solution of the injection. It is usually an immediate side-effect but is not permanent, and the treatment for this is a cold compress.

Following the injection there is also a small risk of developing depigmentation (loss of skin colour) and or/fat atrophy (wasting) around the injection site, the risk of this can vary with different steroid preparations. Some people who have diabetes may find following the injection that their blood sugar levels rise in the first few days and so need to monitor blood sugar levels and adjust diet/ medication accordingly.

Temporary facial flushing may rarely occur following the administration of the steroid injection and there is the potential risk of anaphylaxis (allergic reaction), although this is very rare.

Hyaluronic acid

Hyaluronic acid is a naturally occurring component of the synovial fluid and is also found in the cartilage. It is highly viscous and acts as a shock absorber within the joint, it also stores energy that can be released when there is rapid joint movement and acts as a lubricant when there is slower movement. It is thought that it has a role in maintaining a healthy cartilage. In the osteoarthritic joint there is less naturally occurring hyaluronic acid and it can be less viscous.

By injecting hyaluronic acid directly into the joint the depleted levels are replenished and hence ease the pain and improve function of the joint. The early regime of administering hyaluronic acid was by weekly injections for three to five weeks, although newer preparations require only one or two injections per course.

Who are they suitable for?

Again, most research has been focused on the knee joint and has found this treatment is most beneficial for those with mild to moderate osteoarthritis. It has also been shown that the presence of swelling may predict a poor response to this injection. Further studies are needed to evaluate if they are effective for the hip joint and the shoulder joint, although early indications are that it may be beneficial for osteoarthritis of the shoulder.

How effective are they?

Hyaluronic acid injections are not a cure for osteoarthritis, but they are used to help reduce the symptoms (pain, swelling, stiffness). The benefits are usually noticed between two to five weeks, although this can vary, and flatten out between five to thirteen weeks. The benefits usually last about six months and are similar in magnitude to that of non-steroidal anti-inflammatory drugs.

Safety

Short term there have been no reported complications using hyaluronic acid, but studies are still needed to establish long-term effects of its use and to examine if there are any anatomical benefits/disadvantages. Like all intra-articular injections, there is a small risk of infection in the joint.

Side-effects

Immediately following the injection one can experience increased pain, and up to 10 per cent of people can develop increased pain, swelling and hotness of the joint following the first or second injection. This may vary according to the type of preparation used, but it is thought that this may occur as an immune response to the injection contents and/or due to the technique used, for example the angle of the knee or needle. The side-effects are usually short-lived and treatment usually consists of a cold compress, rest and analgesics.

Conclusion

It is recognized that intra-articular injections can have a role to play in the management of osteoarthritis, in particular of the knee. These injections are used widely in America and in Europe in the management plans of patients who have osteoarthritis.

Corticsteroids are useful for those who have an effusion or flare-up of the pain and who are not able to take NSAIDS. They have a quick onset for symptom relief but they also have a shorter duration period.

Hyaluronic acid injections are useful for those with mild to moderate osteoarthritis, they have a slower onset but a longer duration of action. Unfortunately they are more costly and entail up to five injections at weekly intervals for maximum benefit.

With either of these injections it is important to be treated by a qualified and experienced pracitioner to achieve maximum benefit. It is also important to remember to use them as part of a package including analgesia, pacing, exercising and keeping to a healthy weight.

14

Pacing and maintaining activities

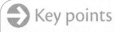 Key points

- Pacing is an important strategy to use in the management of osteoarthritis.

- Pacing does not cost anything!

- Pacing will help us maintain activites without causing unacceptable levels of pain.

- Pacing will enable us to participate in activities that we value.

- On paper pacing seems easy, but in practice it can be challenging.

- Some people who have chronic pain have found pacing to be invaluable.

As we have seen, osteoarthritis can affect people in many ways. For some it can be a minor to moderate inconvenience whilst for others it can have a huge impact on their lifestyle.

When we don't have pain, we find it easy to adapt to life's challenges: housework, travelling to and from work, hobbies, preparing food or going out with friends or family become accepted as everyday activities which can be carried out without too much thought. However, living with long-term pain can be quite different. It becomes more difficult for us to be spontaneous with activities, and everyday chores, let alone activities of enjoyment, become major concerns for individuals.

We know that for many people pain can fluctuate from day to day, or even during the course of the day, whilst for others pain is more constant. It is human nature on good days or at good times of the day for us to try and catch

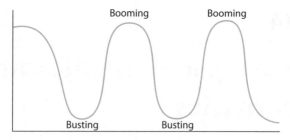

Figure 14.1 A 'boom and busting' activity pattern. High levels of activities are followed by rest to aid recovery.

up with activities, often pushing us to do 'just that little bit more' before stopping. This invariably leads to a period of rest in order to recover. This type of pattern is often called 'boom and busting' – periods of activity followed by periods of down time (Fig 14.1). Other people find that regardless of the pain they keep pushing on through the pain for long periods until a severe flare-up of the pain forces them to stop, often leading to prolonged periods of rest to aid recovery (Fig 14.2). There are other people who avoid most activities each day in an attempt to prevent pain and consequently their activity and fitness levels become extremely poor (Fig 14.3). You may recognize these patterns yourself and find that you are doing one or more of them.

Different patterns of activity

Unfortunately with both the boom and busting and the pushing on approaches, over time the periods of activity become less and the periods of rest and recovery become longer. With these types of activity patterns it is not uncommon

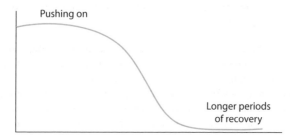

Figure 14.2 The 'pushing on' activity pattern. Carrying on with activities with high levels of pain and without breaks can lead to flare-ups that mean longer periods of rest to aid recovery.

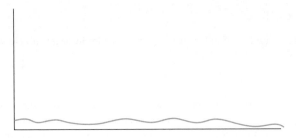

Figure 14.3 'Activity avoidance'. In the hope of avoiding pain very little activity is performed, which unfortunately leads to the opposite of the desired effect and causes reduced fitness, increased stiffness and pain.

for people to stop doing some of the activities that used to be carried out and in so doing creating a low mood, reduced fitness and social isolation. You may recognize yourself that you are now doing less activities than before.

What is pacing?

Pacing is not a cure for osteoarthritis: it is the term used for enabling activities to become more manageable. Pacing is the breaking down of activities into smaller manageable chunks and alternating different types of activity or combining them with periods of rest. The aim of pacing is to ensure daily activity levels are achieved without creating the boom–bust or pushing on scenarios that invariably result in reduced activity and increased pain. By pacing, whether you are having a good day or a bad day, there will be small activities that you can do. Many people who have learned to pace find that they are able to achieve more and more as time goes by and that their flare-ups of the pain are reduced. In many ways pacing is something we should all be doing, whatever age we are.

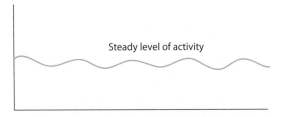

Figure 14.4 'Activity pattern when pacing'. Having a steady level of activity ensures that the pain does not flare, and the need for recovery time is diminished.

How to pace

There are a number of different things to consider in order to help you pace effectively.

Baselines

Establishing your baseline is one of the first things to do. A baseline is the length of time you can do something without it causing pain if your pain is intermittent, or causing an unpleasant level of pain if it is constant. For example if you have OA of the knee, hip or back this may include timing how long you can sit, stand and walk for. If you have OA of the fingers or hand it may include how long you can peel potatoes or knit. If you have OA of the shoulder your baseline may be to see how long you can hold your arm up or drive and so on.

Once taken, you can then use the baselines when carrying out activities and planning your day. For example, if you have OA of the knee and find that your baseline for walking is 10 minutes, ensure that you do not exceed more than a 10-minute walk at any one time, remembering that activities such as pushing the lawnmower or vacuuming are activities that also involve walking. The good thing about baselines is their flexibility. If you find that your 10-minute walk causes or increases your pain, then you can reduce your baseline, similarly if you find your baseline is too low then you can increase it. Remember that your baseline should not be the level that causes or increases your pain, it is the level before the pain starts or increases. If you find your baselines can vary on a good day and bad day (as many people do) then take the lower reading as your baseline as it is always best to start with a low baseline and then increase it, rather than be disillusioned with a baseline you are having problems reaching.

Some therapists have different ways of calculating baselines, but keeping it simple is probably the most effective. As time goes by some people find that their baselines do not change, while others may find they are able to increase this baseline very gradually. Remember, *a baseline is there to stop you pushing yourself into pain.*

Identifying daily and weekly activities

The next step is to examine your daily pattern of activity, often keeping a diary of events and activities is helpful. You may find that you do all your heavy housework in the morning with nothing in the afternoon! It is also important to assess your weekly routine, as you may find that you do all your main walking at one end of the week! By doing this simple task alone you may find you can move activities around and mix and match them: for example you could spread your housework out over the day rather than completing it in one

Table 14.1 A diary to help identify your pattern of daily activity

	Monday	Tuesday	Wednesday	Thursday	Friday	Saturday	Sunday
Rising							
Breakfast							
	Hoover whole house						
	Clean bedrooms and bathrooms						
Lunchtime							
	Food shop						
	Get dinner ready						
	Cut lawns						
Dinner time							
	Pain causes period of recovery						
Bedtime							

morning, or you could complete a small piece of gardening each day as opposed to spending one whole day at it.

Alternating activities

Pacing is about alternating activities down into manageable chunks and mixing different types of activity. All activities involve a range of physical movement, and it is important to recognize which movements are associated with each activity. Below is a list of some of these and next to them are some examples of activities that are associated with them.

♦ Walking (shopping, playing golf, vacuuming).

♦ Standing (ironing, washing-up, preparing food).

♦ Sitting (driving, watching TV, playing cards, reading).

♦ Climbing stairs (at the theatre, on public transport).

♦ Lying down (sunbathing, sleeping, watching TV).

♦ Use of upper arm and shoulder (driving, playing golf, hair styling).

♦ Use of hands (gripping, knitting, cutting and peeling fruit and vegetables).

It would be useful for you to think about the activities you want to carry out and also the type of physical movement it will include. Once you have done this you can then mix up the different types of activities so that no two similar movements are next to each other.

Planning

Some of us are better than others at planning daily and weekly activities; some are very organized whilst others are very erratic and what they do each day is often decided on the hoof, depending on their level of pain at the time. For some an age-old routine has been ingrained in them – washing Monday, shopping Tuesday, and so on. It is helpful to pre-plan your daily and weekly activities, mixing and matching the different types of activity. On closer examination you may find that such ingrained routines are not that helpful. Ensure that you put time aside to plan your day and week and remember to incorporate rest and relaxation into your daily plan.

Incorporating rest

Rest should be incorporated into your day because it is an important part of your management. It is considered healthy if planned and for not too long a period; some recommend five to ten minutes as a good guide. Rest could be sitting down (if standing and walking is a problem to you) or it could mean pulling over at a service station if driving is a problem to you. Rest should be interspersed throughout the day and used in a healthy way. If you are pacing correctly you should not be using rest as a way of relieving your pain.

Relaxation

This should also be incorporated into your daily routine and not be carried out in a last-minute attempt to deal with a pain flare-up. Many people forget to carry out relaxation, but by planning it into your day this is less likely to occur (see Chapter 16 on thoughts and emotions).

Prioritizing

Many of us are familiar with the term 'too many things to do and not enough hours in the day'. Prioritize those things that you need to do versus things that can wait. Make a list of all the things that you want to do in the week then mark off the ones that are important. For instance it may be more important to collect your grandchildren from school than vacuum the spare room! It is helpful to identify those things that need doing today, those things that can wait until the next day and the things that can be done whenever. People find that prioritizing takes the stress away from them.

Problem-solving and compromising

If you find that there are occasions when planning and prioritizing are just not going to help you, then you will have to problem-solve. To do this think of as many different ways to overcome a problem – they may be ridiculous or they may be quite helpful. For instance, if catering for a big group of friends at the end of a week is daunting due to the long periods of weight-bearing, then you could think about eating out, making food in advance and/or freezing food, arranging a take-away or having an easy salad. If going to do the Christmas shopping is worrying you because of the prolonged queuing and walking, then think about choosing a quiet shopping day, choosing an easy shopping mall, getting a taxi there, going with a friend, shopping via the Web or via catalogues.

Whatever your difficulties or worries, think of alternatives. If playing 18 holes of golf is too much then drop down to 9 holes, if doing 9 holes is too much then drop down to 5 and then meet your partner in the bar later. There may not be an easy answer and there may not be a perfect solution, but you may find that you can compromise. By doing this you can still get the job done or achieve some enjoyment from an activity.

For those who like sport and hobbies it can seem like a big loss when the pain stops you from participating. Sometimes changing a hobby or sport to one that is less stressful on the joints may be the solution. Ask yourself what it is about the hobby or the sport that you enjoy: is it the exercise and sport itself, feeling part of a team or is it the regular meeting with friends? Once you have identified the things that you value from activities see if there is a compromise or an alternative solution. You may find that you still get enjoyment going down to watch or coach a local team or by taking part in the management of the local club.

Goal-setting

As mentioned earlier, people often find that they are doing fewer activities than before. This may include daily chores around the home; the discontinuation of hobbies, holidays or being unable to keep up with friends or family. It is often easy to lose sight of the things that both need to do, things that we enjoy doing and the things that we value in our lives.

Goal-setting is all about identifying an activity that you would like to be able to achieve and then establishing a plan as to how to achieve it. Without identifying any goals it is easy to carry on as before, which can have the consequence of missing out on many things in life. So first you need to identify your own goal or goals. Some people choose the following:

- One for around the home, which involves housework or gardening.

- One that is pleasurable, such as a trip to the theatre or a holiday.

- A goal that involves socializing with other people.

Take time to think about what is important in your life. It could be that being able to babysit for the grandchildren is important, playing golf or going to the local bar to have fun again with your friends are the really important things to you. Of course you can always add to your goals to involve more things as time goes by but there a few things to remember when setting your goals:

- *Be specific:* the goal should be very specific. For instance, rather than just improve walking, your goal could be to walk in the forest for a picnic or to go shopping with the grandchildren to buy their birthday present.

- *Be meaningful:* the goals need to be meaningful to you – they should be your own goals and not ones that your family think you should do!

- *Achievable:* the goals should be ones that you yourself feel are achievable within a realistic time frame. Not doing this could lead to failing and huge disappointments.

◆ *Be realistic:* the goals need to be realistic: for example, returning to university at the age of 80 with the goal of going into space may not be very realistic!

◆ *Time:* you should set yourself a realistic timescale or things may never get done!

It helps to write down your goals and then plan how you are going to achieve them by breaking them down into small chunks. It is here that the baselines play a role, as they are a true indicator of what your current limits of comfort are for different activities. If your goal were to go and see a cricket or baseball match you would need to plan the trip. How much walking would it entail? How much sitting? What about drinks and visiting rest rooms? What about climbing stairs? Would you drive or go on public transport? Like many goals there are often many different factors to consider; this is not to say that it is unachievable. These factors were always there, but before you had osteoarthritis they were often insignificant to you. Once you have broken the goal down into small chunks you can see the things that you may need to practice beforehand or things that you need to organize.

What makes pacing so difficult?

Although on paper pacing seems very straightforward, many people find it is difficult to put into practice due to several common factors.

Habits

Habits are things that we do automatically without really thinking about it. Some habits are very important and serve a useful purpose, for instance putting the seat belt on in the car will stop an injury during an emergency stop and cleaning your teeth at night prevents tooth decay developing. However, there are also many habits that we all have which on closer examination serve no real important purpose in the larger scheme of things, for instance moving all the heavy furniture every time you want to vacuum or completing all the washing on one day of the week.

Many people find that when they start to pace, some of these habits can get in the way. Ask yourself, is it a useful habit? Why do I do it like this? Can I change it and still get the same result? By problem-solving and changing a habit you may find it possible to pace and still achieve what you set out to do.

Expectations

We all have standards and expectations which we strive for, and some people find that pacing can challenge this. Compromising has already been mentioned and although it makes sense in some situations it is not always easy to follow through. Some people feel that it may seem like giving in to things or that they are settling for second best. It is important to ask yourself if the activity in hand is worth pushing into the pain barrier which may cause a flare-up of your pain.

Time

We all live in a busy world today with work, friends and family, and breaking your activities down into manageable chunks may make you feel you will never get a job done. It is true that the completion of a task may take a little longer than previously, but you will be able to complete more at a steady level as opposed to the boom–bust pattern. Traffic controllers on busy roadways have two choices during rush hour, they can either let people speed at the maximum rates, which causes queues and stoppages, or they can get the traffic to flow at a slower steady rate, which allows a free flow of traffic. The outcome is that the journey may take the same length of time but those in the second scenario will be less stressed.

Family and friends

You may find that some of your friends and family find it frustrating watching you breaking things down into small chunks and may intervene and try and take over, some may even become impatient and so put extra pressure on you to either push on into pain or give in altogether. Changing your routines and habits can affect those around you. The answer to this is to let them know that you are trying to pace, and inform them that by doing this you are more likely to complete activities without increasing the pain. In so doing it is hoped they will allow you to continue with a task in your own time.

Conclusion

Pacing is widely taught in the field of pain management and it has been shown to be highly effective in helping people maintain daily activities without pushing into unacceptable levels of pain or causing long periods of rest. Identifying goals and then using the pacing technique helps us all to continue with the activities that we personally value.

Pacing can be used effectively on its own, but it is also important to use it in conjunction with the other strategies for managing pain, such as medication or injections, as it enhances the effects of the treatments.

15

Device use and other therapies

Heat and cold

The decision to use either heat or cold should be discussed with your doctor or physiotherapist. Moist heat, such as a warm bath or shower, or dry heat, such as a heating pad, placed on the painful area of the joint for about 15 minutes may relieve the pain. An ice pack (or a bag of frozen vegetables) wrapped in a towel and placed on the sore area for about 15 minutes may help to reduce swelling and stop the pain. If you have poor circulation, do not use cold packs.

Transcutaneous electrical nerve stimulation

A small transcutaneous electrical nerve stimulation (TENS) device that directs mild electric pulses to nerve endings that lie beneath the skin in the painful area may relieve some arthritis pain. TENS seems to work by producing high-frequency electrical stimulation of the nerve, which disrupts pain messages to the brain, and by modifying pain perception.

Ambulatory assist devices

Consider a cane, used in the hand opposite the painful joint, in patients with persistent walking pain from hip or knee OA. A cane reduces loading force on the joint and is associated with a decrease in pain in patients with hip and knee OA. If you have OA in both legs (not just one) then it may be preferable to use a walker/frame to distribute load evenly.

To use this stand comfortably and erect with your weight evenly balanced on your walker. Move your walker forward a short distance. Then move forward,

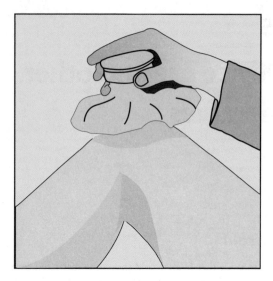

Figure 15.1 Application of heat or ice to an affected area can greatly facilitate pain relief.

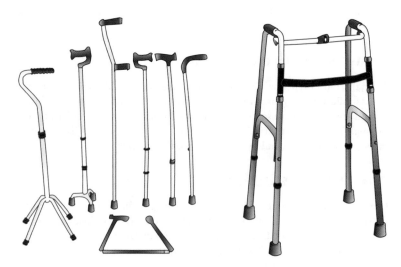

Figure 15.2 Walking sticks, canes, crutches and a walking frame.

lifting your leg so that the heel of your foot will touch the floor first. As you move, your knee and ankle will bend and your entire foot will rest evenly on the floor. As you complete the step allow your toe to lift off the floor. Move the walker again and your knee and hip will again reach forward for your next step. Remember, touch your heel first, then flatten your foot, then lift your toes off the floor. Try to walk as smoothly as you can. Don't hurry.

Walking sticks, canes and crutches should be available through consulting an occupational therapist, visiting a medical device store and frequently can also be found in pharmacies.

Knee braces

The importance of mechanical factors in the development of OA may explain why knee OA occurs more often in the medial (inner) compartment, presumably due to its increased loading during gait. Despite the apparent important role of mechanics in the development of knee osteoarthritis, few therapies have attempted to relieve the forces responsible for disease. Two therapies that have attempted to modify these forces are knee braces and heel wedges.

Since involvement of the medial compartment is especially frequent, interventions whose goal is to realign the knee so as to reduce loading on

Laternal heel wedge

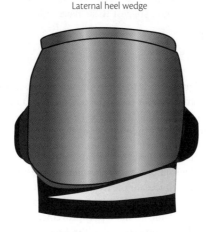

Right shoe

Figure 15.3 A lateral heel wedge.

the medial compartment, such as valgus bracing, are used clinically. For those with instability of the knee, there is evidence that valgus bracing and orthotic devices shifts the load away from the medial compartment, and, in doing so, may provide considerable relief of pain and improvement in function.

Wedged insoles

One way of lessening load across the medial compartment would be to insert an insole into the shoe that alters the distribution of load in the foot which in turn alters load at the knee. In particular, lateral wedge insoles (lateral aspect higher than medial) increase hindfoot valgus in an attempt to straighten out the leg, and produce less medial knee loading.

Japanese investigators have invented and tested such a 'wedged insole' for treatment of medial osteoarthritis and have suggested that when wedged insoles are used, there is an increasing valgus angulation of the calcaneus (turning out the heel) that produces a more upright leg with less medial knee loading.

The symptomatic effect of wedged insoles has been evaluated in a number of uncontrolled studies and more recently in controlled trials. The earlier studies suggested that wedges provided short-term symptomatic benefit. The randomized controlled trial showed a reduction in NSAID (anti-inflammatory) consumption in the insole treated group. Despite some supportive evidence, the strongest evidence would suggest these have little if any impact on osteoarthritis pain.

Valgus bracing

The concept of a valgus brace is to apply, during weight-bearing, a moment to the knee, which directly opposes the usual damaging moment and thus reduces load on the inner compartment. Figure 15.4 shows one of the examples of a valgus brace on a right leg which functions through three-point bending.

A number of biomechanical studies have demonstrated an improvement in many aspects of gait with valgus (knock-kneed) bracing in knee OA. Some studies of the effectiveness of unloader braces for the treatment of varus (bow legged) knee OA have also been reported. These studies demonstrate that wearing a valgus brace gives a clinically significant and immediate improvement in the pain and function of patients with medial osteoarthritis of the knee. The valgus brace group

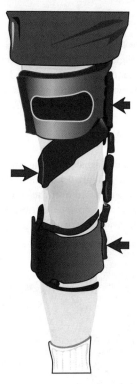

Figure 15.4 External abduction moment applied by a medial hinge brace, which can 'push' the knee into valgus.

significantly reduced their pain by approximately 50 per cent at 12 weeks and this was maintained at 24 weeks. To put this improvement in symptoms into context, most studies of anti-inflammatories suggest they relieve about 15–20 per cent of pain. Newer brace designs may facilitate greater compliance as currently the efficacy of braces is limited to the time for which they are worn – they were often large, bulky and difficult to wear under clothes, so adherence to their use has been a problem. Despite this they appear very effective for pain and the newer brace designs may overcome many of the shortcomings of older brace technology.

Patella taping

Physiotherapists tape the knee as short-term or intermittent treatment for knee pain. Knee taping (Figure 15.5) is believed to relieve pain by improving alignment of the patellofemoral joint and/or unloading inflamed soft tissues. A recent trial found that therapeutic taping of the knee is effective in the management of pain and disability in patients with OA.

Braces for the hand

Splinting of the first carpometacarpal joint (the base of the thumb), preferably with prefabricated neoprene (Figure 15.6), can be facilitated by an occupational therapist or possibly purchased over the counter. The thumb splint can be worn full-time until an acute episode settles, or alternatively only worn during performance of aggravating activities.

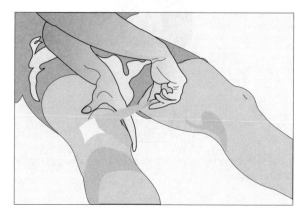

Figure 15.5 The application of patella taping has been shown to improve symptoms in knee osteoarthritis.

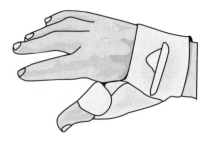

Figure 15.6 A hand brace.

16

Thoughts and emotions

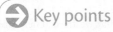 Key points

- Thoughts and emotions play a part in our everyday lives.

- It is natural for people with osteoarthritis to have some negative thoughts which may cause anxiety and occasionally depression.

- Anxiety and depression can be successfully addressed with an array of treatments.

- If these emotions are not addressed it becomes more difficult to manage the osteoarthritis.

The one thing that we have in common is that we all experience thoughts and emotions in our daily life. These thoughts and emotions can be both negative and positive, and are part of the way we process events in our lives. There are many thoughts and feelings that we can experience when diagnosed with a chronic condition such as osteoarthritis. Thoughts such as: why me? why can't I be cured?, will I end up in a wheelchair? how will I cope? These can create unhelpful emotions such as anger, fear and worry. We can feel frustrated at not being able to do some simple tasks, grieve at losing hobbies and interests and feel guilty asking others to help with chores, sometimes resulting in a feeling of helplessness or worthlessness.

For some people these thoughts and feelings are normal responses to receiving the news that they have osteoarthritis. For many they are not ongoing and so do not play a major role in their lives. However, for some people these thoughts and feelings can persist and in so doing, become more unhelpful and impact on the way osteoarthritis is managed and also increase the pain experience. Our thoughts and feelings are as important as the disease process itself and should not be seen as a weakness.

What are thoughts?

Throughout our day when we are engaged with something, our brain is having thoughts. A thought can be described as something we are saying in our head, for example 'I think they like me', 'the chocolate cake looks delicious', 'do I look fat in this'! Thoughts can be both negative and positive in their nature and affect the way we feel about ourselves.

What are emotions?

Emotions (feelings) are the result of the thoughts that we have. There are many different negative and positive emotions that we can experience for example: joy, happiness, sadness, fear, worry, anger and jealousy are just a few. You may feel elated if they like you, or feel guilty eating the chocolate cake.

Behaviours

Our feelings affect the way that we behave: for example, if the thoughts on going to the dentist are positive – he will make my teeth white – then we are more likely to go on a regular basis for check-ups. However, if the thought of the dentist's chair causes a feeling of fear then our behaviour may be quite different, you may only go when you get severe toothache!

How thoughts, emotions and behaviour are related

Thoughts affect our emotions, which affect our behaviour. The way we behave then affects our thought process and so a vicious cycle starts (Fig.16.1).

Common thoughts and emotions when diagnosed with osteoarthritis

For some people the diagnosis of osteoarthritis can be a relief: 'I thought I had a life-threatening condition', 'people will understand now why I have the pain'. However, for many in the early stages following the diagnosis of osteoarthritis, there are unhelpful emotions of anger, denial and worry.

Anger

People can be angry for various reasons: we can feel angry that we have the condition and that there is no cure, angry with the doctors, angry that we cannot pursue interests and hobbies, and angry that the osteoarthritis is intruding in our lives.

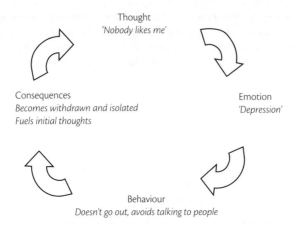

Thought
'Nobody likes me'

Consequences
Becomes withdrawn and isolated
Fuels initial thoughts

Emotion
'Depression'

Behaviour
Doesn't go out, avoids talking to people

Figure 16.1 Common thoughts and emotions when diagnosed with osteoarthritis.

Denial

Initially we can deny that we have osteoarthritis – 'it only happens to others', or 'I think this is something else'. As time goes by this denial makes it difficult to put management strategies into place. If left it can lead to reduced functioning.

Worry

There are many concerns and questions that people have when first diagnosed with osteoarthritis. 'Will it get worse?', 'I will not be able to manage'.

Depression and anxiety

If these unhelpful thoughts mentioned above are not addressed they can lead to more unhelpful emotions such as depression and anxiety. These two emotions are well recognized in many people who are living with a chronic condition such as osteoarthritis. There are also some people who have depression and anxiety prior to this diagnosis.

Depression and osteoarthritis

The type of depression that we shall discuss here is unipolar, as opposed to bipolar depression (manic depression). Unfortunately depression is still a condition that people do not like to talk about, but this is not to say that it is not common. It is thought that 19 per cent of the general population have depression and that up to one-third of people who have osteoarthritis have some degree of depression: it is therefore a relatively common condition seen by doctors. Research has shown that if you experienced depression before the age of 40 then you are more likely to experience depression again with the onset of chronic pain, such as that experienced in osteoarthritis.

What are the signs and symptoms?

It is part of human nature to have good days and low days, but this alone does not lead to a diagnosis of depression: it is thought that 65 per cent of the population experience low mood at some time in their life. Most of us will probably recall a time in the past two weeks of feeling 'fed up' for a short time and some would say it is an essential part of our make-up to have some lows in our lives in order for us to experience the highs!

Depression, like pain, is a very personal experience to each individual but generally consists of a persistent unpleasant feeling of despair and sadness. The severity can vary from mild where the person can experience feelings of down-heartedness, to severe where the person can lose all confidence, have no self-worth and have thoughts of wanting to end life. Health professionals will diagnose depression if:

◆ You have been feeling low in your mood and/or have lost interest and pleasure in things every day for the past two weeks PLUS:

  Four of the following symptoms most days, over the past two weeks:

  ◆ Feeling of fatigue and loss of energy (loss of motivation to carry out enjoyable tasks, daytime sleeping).

  ◆ Unable to sleep at night, and/or early waking (not due to pain) or excessive sleeping during the day.

  ◆ Irritability (snappy with friends and family).

  ◆ Reduced concentration or inability to make decisions (could be a work or at home).

  ◆ Loss or increase of appetite or weight (weight loss, comfort eating).

  ◆ Feelings of excessive guilt or worthlessness ('I am not a good parent', 'I can't do anything').

  ◆ Morbid thoughts (suicidal or self-harming thoughts).

If you feel having read this list that you have the symptoms of depression then it is important to go and discuss it further with your doctor.

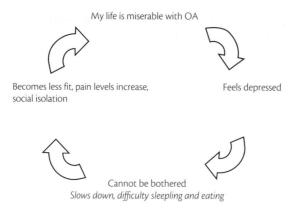

My life is miserable with OA

Becomes less fit, pain levels increase,
social isolation

Feels depressed

Cannot be bothered
Slows down, difficulty sleepling and eating

Figure 16.2 The effects of depression on osteoarthritis.

The effects of depression on osteoarthritis

As mentioned above, our thoughts and feelings affect our behaviour. If left untreated, depression can increase the amount of pain and discomfort we feel as a result of osteoarthritis and can affect the way we manage our lives. Figure 16.2 demonstrates this.

It is important to recognize and treat depression and to break this vicious circle. Having depression is not a sign of weakness, it is a normal reaction to an unwanted situation, such as being told that you have osteoarthritis.

Anxiety

What is anxiety?

Anxiety is a natural human response to certain situations. Many of us experience anxiety when visiting the dentist, parents experience a certain amount of anxiety when watching their children reciting at a school concert, and soldiers feel anxious before going into battle. Anxiety is a natural protective mechanism that prepares our body for dangerous or uncomfortable situations where we may need to fight or flee (stay and confront or run away). It is thought that this stems back to the days when survival was an everyday part of life: physiological changes were necessary to help us run from a lion, or wolf, or to fight with bears!

Anxiety itself is therefore not a problem, as it helps us to survive and deal with certain situations. However, it can become troublesome when there is no longer an imminent danger present, but you still feel anxious and experience the symptoms of anxiety. Specific types of anxiety which include phobias, panic attacks and general anxiety disorders require specialist treatment and will not be discussed in this book.

The signs and symptoms of anxiety

When we experience anxiety in response to a perceived threat our body releases a hormone called adrenalin. Adrenalin has many actions on different parts of the body with the aim of preparing us for fight or flight. Physical symptoms of anxiety can be identified in Figure 16.3.

Anxiety and osteoarthritis

It is not uncommon for anxious people to expect the worse, worry about things before they happen, and worry that they will not be able to cope. The worrying thoughts of those who have osteoarthritis, including 'why me' and 'I wont be able to cope', can lead to unacceptable levels of anxiety. Such thoughts cause the body to jump into action and release adrenalin and then the body

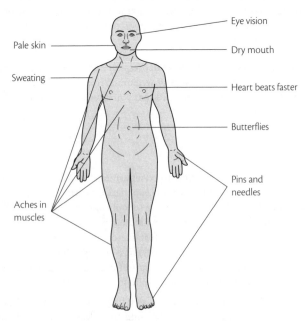

Figure 16.3 The physical effects that anxiety can have on the body.

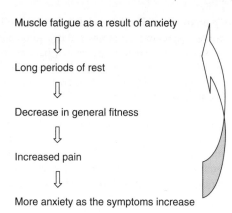

Muscle fatigue as a result of anxiety

⇩

Long periods of rest

⇩

Decrease in general fitness

⇩

Increased pain

⇩

More anxiety as the symptoms increase

Figure 16.4 The effects of anxiety on osteoarthritis.

develops the symptoms of anxiety. For people who have long-term pain due to osteoarthritis the physical affects of anxiety are very unhelpful.

Treatment for depression and anxiety

There are treatments and things that you can do yourself to help manage these unhelpful thoughts and feelings. The different types of treatment consist of:

- Education.

- Medication.

- Counselling.

- Cognitive behaviour therapy.

- Relaxation.

Ideally, combinations of treatments work best. It is important to discuss the available treatments with your doctor, who is skilled at identifying your level of anxiety and or depression and will know what would be the best treatment plan.

Education

It has been shown that the more information we have about a chronic condition the more successful we are at managing it. People with osteoarthritis who suffer from depression or anxiety can benefit greatly from health professionals who provide information on the condition. It is helpful to understand what osteoarthritis is, how it develops, signs and symptoms and its natural progression. This can help deal with some of the anxieties that we may have. Some centres offer clinics and helplines with the aim of providing information about all aspects of osteoarthritis. Some of these educational sessions are held in groups whilst others are offered on a one-to-one basis.

In some areas, you may have access to pain-management programmes, which deal with the management of chronic pain conditions, including osteoarthritis. These programmes are run by a team of different health professionals and address thoughts and feelings as key components in managing pain. They are geared to managing the pain as opposed to curing it, and have been shown to be beneficial.

The Internet has opened up a whole new source of information. There are several websites available regarding osteoarthritis, which can provide useful information. It should be said, however, that clinicians recommend that these websites are chosen with caution as some can be misleading or inaccurate. You will find some useful addresses at the end of this book. Information regarding osteoarthritis can also be gained from recognized groups such as the ARC (Arthritis Research Campaign) and OARSI (Osteoarthritis Research Society International). These provide very accurate and useful leaflets and contacts.

Antidepressants for depression and anxiety

For moderate to severe depression, medication is recommended. They can be very effective in up to 70 per cent of people who have depression, but like many medications used to treat medical conditions, it may take a while to find the right drug for each individual at the correct dose. There are three main groups of antidepressant medications available on prescription and these are shown in Table 16.1.

Your doctor will discuss with you the most suitable antidepressant, taking into account your past and current medical history, and other medications that you are taking. All antidepressant medicines should be prescribed by a qualified doctor who has knowledge of the contraindications, interactions and potential side-effects.

Tricyclics

Tricyclics (TCAs) have been on the market in England for over 30 years and have been shown to be useful to help treat depression and anxiety. They are also used at lower doses to treat chronic pain.

Table 16.1

Tricyclics (TCAs)	Amitriptyline hydrochloride
	Amoxapine
	Clomipramine hydrochloride
	Dosulepin hydrochloride
	Doxepin
	Imipramine
	Lofepramine
	Nortriptyline
	Trimipramine
Closely related to tricyclics	Maprotiline hydrochloride
	Mianserin hydrochloride
	Trazodone hydrochloride
Selective serotonin reuptake inhibitors (SSRIs)	Citalopram
	Escitalopram
	Fluoxetine
	Fluvoxamine
	Sertraline
Monoamine oxidase inhibitors (MAOIs) and reversible inhibitors of monomine oxidase (RIMAs)	Isocarboxazid
	Phenelzine
	Tranylcypromine
Other antidepressant drugs	Flupentixol
	Mirtazapine
	Reboxetine
	Tryptophan
	Venlafaxine

Selective serotonin reuptake inhibitors

Selective serotonin reuptake inhibitors (SSRIs) have been on the market for the past 15 years. They are also used in the treatment of anxiety and some specific disorders such as anorexia, obsessive–compulsive disorder and panic attacks. They are becoming increasingly popular in the management of depression and anxiety.

Monoamine oxidase inhibitors

Monoamine oxidase inhibitors (MOAIs) are an older type of medication. They are effective for all types of depression but are usually only used in severe cases of depression. Unfortunately MAOIs carry unwanted side-effects and can interact dangerously with certain foods, hence they are not so popular now.

 Questions and answers about antidepressants

Q 1. How soon will it take for them to help my mood?

A.   In the majority of people the depression may not improve for about 2–3 weeks although in elderly people this may take up to 6–8 weeks. Some people can report feeling worse before seeing the benefits and for this reason it is important for anyone starting an anti-depressant to be regularly reviewed by a clinician or nurse.

Q 2. How long will I have to take them?

A.   For those who have not had depression previously, it is recommended that the medication is continued for approximately 4–6 months following an improvement in the symptoms, with a view to preventing future relapses. For those who have had depression previously or with recurrent depression, your doctor may recommend the antidepressants are taken for a longer period of time. It is important to discuss the likely duration of treatment with your doctor at the start of your treatment.

Q 3. Do they have side-effects?

A.   Yes, like many medicines there can be side-effects, however they vary from drug to drug, and from person to person. Your doctor should discuss this with you before starting treatment. It is important to seek advice should you experience unwanted side-effects. Some people find that it takes a trial of more than one tablet before finding the one that is best suited. Individual side-effects of each drug will not be discussed here so it is important to discuss them with your doctor.

Q 4. Will I become addicted to them?

A.   It is not uncommon for people to be reluctant to take recommended medication for depression due to fears of addiction. Current advice is that antidepressant drugs are not addictive, however if stopped abruptly some people find they develop 'discontinuation symptoms' which may include headaches and nausea. For this reason it would be advisable for you to seek medical advice if planning to stop the medication. It is good practice for all people taking regular medication to be reviewed by their doctor on a regular basis, as you would do if you had diabetes or hypertension.

Q 5. What is St John's Wort (*Hypericum perforatum*)?

A. This is a herbal remedy that has been popular in recent years for treating mild to moderate depression. However, there are concerns that it can interact with other medications, therefore it is wise to consult your doctor prior to commencing it. St John's Wort should not be taken with prescribed antidepressants and although it can be bought at herbal shops it is important to note that the compositional strength can vary.

Counselling

Some people may find seeing a non-medical counsellor beneficial, particularly if there are other reasons as to why emotions such as depression and anxiety are experienced. As we get older we are more likely to encounter bereavements, or families moving away resulting in isolation. These are situations that can contribute to low moods Your GP will be able to recommend a recognized counsellor in your area.

Cognitive behaviour therapy

If your clinician feels that your levels of anxiety or depression are severe and highly distressing in your life then they may refer you on to a cognitive behavioural therapist CBT (a psychologist, nurse, or doctor). Cognitive behaviour therapy is about changing the way that we think (cognitive) in order to alter the way that we behave (behaviour), or vice versa. As mentioned earlier, thoughts and feelings that we have every day affect the way that we behave and a cycle can start. The aim of CBT is to break this cycle so that we have more positive thoughts, which then lead to a more useful behaviour. It sounds very easy on paper, but CBT psychologists and specialist nurses are highly qualified, and spend many years training in this field.

Relaxation

If we refer back to the physical symptoms of anxiety, it includes muscle tension which in turn leads to muscle fatigue and increased pain levels. The aim of relaxation is to therefore break this cycle by relaxing the muscle tension, enabling the body to recharge itself.

Can everyone do it?

Most people are able to practise relaxation, however there are some people for whom it may not be recommended, for instance those who have low blood pressure or cardiac conditions, those with severe depression or who have a history of psychotic hallucinations and delusion. Check with your clinician if you are in doubt.

Deep breathing (diaphragmatic)

The first thing to think about is your breathing. Breathing is obviously a vital bodily function and usually we do not notice the action. However, on closer examination many of us breathe only using the upper part of the lungs rather than the lower part. Unfortunately pain and feeling anxious can make our breathing shallower, which can exacerbate stressful feelings. It is therefore vital to practise deep breathing on a regular basis throughout the day.

How to deep breathe

- Sit comfortably in your chair in an upright position.
- Put your hands on the area below the ribs and above your abdomen.
- Breathe out, then take a longer breath in gently in through the nose.
- You should feel the lower part of the lungs fill with air.
- Your abdomen will move under your hand.
- Hold the breath for a short moment then breath out slowly and fully.
- The breathing can then be repeated.

Many people are surprised how shallow their breathing has become!

Types of relaxation

There are different forms of relaxation available and they range from quick and simple to longer, more involved forms. Some techniques are more physical in their approach (progressive muscle relaxation) and deal with reducing muscle spasm and tension, others are more psychological and help with our thoughts (guided imagery).

Progressive muscle relaxation

There are two different types of muscle:

1. *Involuntary* such as the heart or eye muscles which automatically tense and relaxes.

2. *Voluntary* such as the calf and shoulders muscles which we can decide to tense or relax.

The aim of progressive muscle relaxation (PMR) is to help you recognize those voluntary muscles that are tense and then relax them. As is often the case, we are unaware of muscle tension until we start to explore it.

♦ Tense the muscle for up to 7 seconds and then relaxes it for about 25 seconds.

♦ Tense the muscle by approximately 60 per cent (more than this could cause increased pain).

♦ It is often a good idea to start at the extremities and work your way up the body relaxing and tensing one voluntary muscle at a time (not all at the same time!). For instance, start at the feet and work up through the legs and then the arms and work up to the neck.

Following practice many people discover they can identify when they are tense and then relax the muscle.

Guided imagery

This type of relaxation is popular with many people. It can be likened to having a nice dream. The idea is for you to think of a nice place – at the beach or in a meadow, for example, wherever you feel at ease – and then for you to spend some time in that place. You identify smells and sounds and colours. This guided imagery can take as little or as long as you wish, but it should be a pleasant experience.

Distraction therapy

Listening to chosen music, reading a good book and watching a film are all forms of distraction therapy. They act by diverting our attention away from the pain or the negative feelings.

Check list for successful relaxation

♦ Do your own research into different types of relaxation and then choose the ones that you feel best suit you. Use tapes and books and CDs to help you.

◆ Choose a range of relaxation styles, for example one you could use on the bus that perhaps takes just a few minutes to do or even seconds and then one that you could do in your coffee break, which may take 10 minutes, and then one that lasts 30–40 minutes. By having a range of relaxation techniques you will always have one you can use in different situations.

◆ Relaxation is not easy, *keep practising the different techniques* and they will become easier.

◆ Ensure you have a private room where you can do your longer relaxation and ensure you have a comfortable chair or bed.

◆ Ensure you are not disturbed.

◆ Get into a habit with your relaxation and include it in your everyday routine.

◆ During the day remember to take regular breaks for relaxation. Try not to wait until things become stressful before you do your relaxation – try to pre-empt stress.

Conclusion

Helpful and unhelpful thoughts and feelings play a part in our everyday lives. For those who have a chronic condition such osteoarthritis, negative thoughts can become overwhelming, change our behaviour and inhibit the way we manage the condition. When assessing each patient good clinicians will always ask about worries, anxieties and moods, and offer help where it is needed. Although nobody wants to have osteoarthritis, life can still have fun and enjoyment included in it.

It is important to remember that you are not alone in having some of these negative feelings, and that there are some successful treatments and interventions available today.

17

Surgery

Key Points

♦ If conservative treatments have not been successful and you experience pain and limited motion then surgery may be a therapeutic option for your osteoarthritis.

♦ Complications are frequent and the postoperative rehabilitation process is often lengthy – please give the decision to have surgery appropriate consideration.

Introduction

While most people with osteoarthritis won't need surgery, it might be an option for you if you experience severe joint damage, extreme pain or very limited motion as a result of your OA and other more conservative treatments have been unsuccessful. The decision to use surgery depends on several things including your level of disability, the intensity of pain, the interference with your lifestyle, your age, other health problems and your occupation. Currently, more than 80 per cent of the surgeries performed for osteoarthritis involve replacing the hip or knee joint. An orthopaedic surgeon (a doctor who specializes in surgery on bones and joints) can assist you in determining if surgery is necessary to relieve the pain from osteoarthritis.

Surgery may be performed to:

♦ Remove loose pieces of bone and cartilage from the joint if they are causing mechanical symptoms of buckling or locking.

♦ Resurface (smooth out) bones.

◆   Reposition bones (osteotomy).

◆   Replace joints.

The benefits of surgery include improved movement, pain relief and improved joint alignment. Of course, there are always risks to surgery, especially if you have other health problems or you are overweight, which can add stress to the heart and lungs during surgery. There also is the risk of forming blood clots in your legs.

If you are thinking about having surgery for your osteoarthritis there may be lots of questions on your mind. This chapter aims to provide the most up-to-date information on the options available and to answer the questions which people most often ask, such as: when to have surgery? what surgical options there are? what complications may arise?

When should I have surgery?

Surgery should be resisted when symptoms can be managed by other treatment modalities. If your function and mobility remains compromised despite maximal medical therapy (this includes non-medicinal approaches such as weight loss, exercise and bracing as well as medicinal approaches such as taking analgesics), and if your joint is structurally unstable, you should be considered for surgical intervention. If your pain has progressed to unacceptable levels—that is, pain at rest and/or night-time pain—you should also be considered a surgical candidate. Thus the typical indications for surgery are debilitating pain and major limitation of functions such as walking and daily activities, or impaired ability to sleep or work despite other therapy.

You are an ideal surgical candidate if you have not yet developed appreciable muscle weakness, generalized or cardiovascular deconditioning (loss of bodily and heart function) and you can medically withstand the stress of surgery. To ensure the best return of joint function after surgery, surgery should be performed before your arthritis causes complications such as marked muscle loss. Furthermore, before undergoing surgery you should be in the best possible physical condition and be prepared for rehabilitation after surgery. Full functional recovery after surgery may not be realistically expected if you have significant cognitive impairment, such as dementia, or symptomatic cardiac (heart) or lung disease, since these conditions can impede postoperative rehabilitation.

What surgical options are there?

There are several different types of joint surgery. We discuss below those most commonly used for people with osteoarthritis.

Arthroscopic treatment

Arthroscopy, or 'scoping' a joint, is an outpatient procedure that is used to examine and sometimes repair joints. For arthroscopy, the doctor inserts a viewing tube (an arthroscope) through a small cut (about 5 mm or ¼ in) into the fluid-filled space in the affected joint. The technique can be used to help with diagnosis or to carry out treatment or keyhole surgery using miniaturized instruments.

In arthroscopic debridement the surgeon clears away debris and smooths damaged cartilage in the knee. The role of this type of arthroscopic surgery of the knee for osteoarthritis is controversial. In a well-designed placebo controlled trial of this form of surgery, improvement in symptoms could be attributed to a placebo effect (Moseley *et al.* 2002). The participants in this trial who had real arthroscopic treatment and joint irrigation were compared to others who had a sham procedure. Those who had the sham surgery were taken to the operating room, the doctor simulated arthroscopic surgery, but only nicked the skin and splashed salt-water around to imitate joint irrigation. The amount of improvement was about the same in those who had real arthroscopy when compared to those who got the sham surgery.

However, for a subgroup of knees with loose bodies or flaps of meniscus (disc of cartilage in the knee) or cartilage that are causing mechanical symptoms, especially locking, or catching of the joint, arthroscopic removal of these unstable tissues may improve joint function and alleviate some of these mechanical symptoms. Although this surgery may provide temporary relief of symptoms, it does not stop the progression of arthritis. Thus a selected group of patients with osteoarthritis may benefit from arthroscopy. However, if there is already a lot of osteoarthritis, it may be better to do another type of surgery rather than arthroscopy.

Arthroscopic debridement (clearing away debris and smoothing the cartilage in the knee) is still one of the most common types of surgery performed in people with knee osteoarthritis. In the absence of locking or catching symptoms this surgery will be as effective as taking a placebo (such as a sugar pill). You are still placed at risk of operative complications such as infections and leg clots. If this surgery is offered to you by your surgeon please question its true benefits for management of your symptoms, and balance these against the real risks of operative complications (discussed later in this chapter).

Osteotomy/realignment

Surgery may be used to realign bones and other joint structures that have become misaligned because of long-standing osteoarthritis. For the knee, such

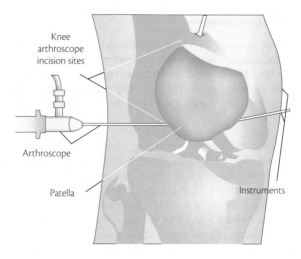

Knee
arthroscope
incision sites

Arthroscope

Patella

Instruments

Figure 17.1 Typical incision sites for knee arthroscopy.

realignment may shift weight-bearing to healthier cartilage where the joint has been unevenly damaged by the osteoarthritis, with resulting pain relief. The procedure is done to relieve stress on the cartilage and prevent further damage to the joint. During an osteotomy, the surgeon removes a small wedge of bone near the affected joint. Removing the piece of bone realigns the bone and improves the contact between the remaining, healthy areas of cartilage in the joint. The tibial osteotomy for the knee may be recommended for a younger, active patient instead of joint replacement surgery.

A recent review of osteotomy suggested that this intervention leads to improvements in pain and function (Brouwer *et al.* 2005). Recovery is typically prolonged, but osteotomy may delay the need for total joint replacement for 5–10 years (Naudie *et al.* 1999). This may allow a knee replacement to be postponed, but it can also make the subsequent replacement of your knee more difficult if a knee replacement were to be needed later on. Currently there is debate as to the relative merits of osteotomy versus unicompartmental knee replacement (single compartment – see the later section on arthoplasty/joint replacement) (Stukenborg-Colsman *et al.* 2001).

Arthrodesis/fusion

A surgical procedure called arthrodesis, or joint fusion, is sometimes used to correct severe joint problems caused by osteoarthritis. In this procedure, the surgeon makes the affected joint permanently immobile by using a bone graft

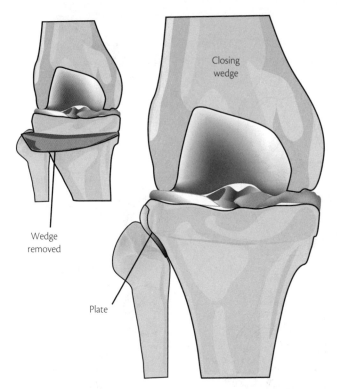

Figure 17.2 The knee during osteotomy with removal of wedge (top left) and after closure with application of plate.

and inserting metal screws, plates, and rods to hold the joint in place. Arthrodesis is performed only when the pain from osteoarthritis is so severe that immobilizing the joint is an improvement. This may be recommended for badly damaged joints for which joint replacement surgery is not appropriate. Fusion may be recommended for joints of the wrist and ankle and the small joints of fingers and toes but is rarely recommended for knees or hips. Joint immobility in large joints such as the knee and hip leads to marked impairments in function and should be avoided unless this procedure is absolutely necessary.

Cartilage grafting/transplantation

Unlike bone, cartilage that is injured does not rejuvenate. Surgery may be used to graft new cartilage cells into damaged regions of cartilage. The benefits of

159

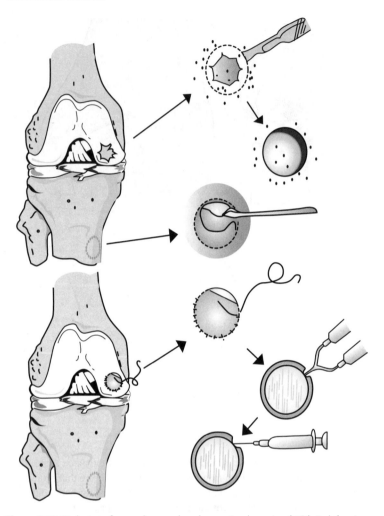

Figure 17.3 Technique for autologous chondrocyte implantation (ACI). A defect is prepared so that it is surrounded by normal, healthy cartilage. A small flap of soft tissue (periosteum) is removed from the tibia to be used as a cover flap. This periosteum is sewn over the defect, and treated with a sealant (fibrin) to avoid leakage of injected cells. Cartilage precursor cells (chondrocytes at an earlier stage of development) harvested at a previous surgery and grown for six weeks (called 'chondrocytes') are injected beneath the flap.

cartilage grafting in arthritic joints is still being studied. Cartilage grafting is likely to be most practical when the cartilage damage is confined to a very small area that is surrounded by normal cartilage. Current techniques are not helpful for people with large areas of thin or absent cartilage, as is typically the case in osteoarthritis.

Cartilage transplantation uses live cells from donated cartilage. This process is known as autologous chondrocyte therapy (ACT) or autologous chondrocyte implantation (ACI). Another technique, called mosaicplasty, involves moving cartilage and some bone from another part of the knee to repair the damaged surface. Graft procedures combining these two techniques may be used to cover larger areas of joint damage. The donated cartilage must be transplanted within 72 hours. The risks of bleeding and joint infection following surgery are probably similar to those with joint replacement. Both mosaicplasty and ACT/ACI may be more widely used in the future, though it is not possible to be certain of this yet, and their role in management of osteoarthritis today is limited. As mentioned, they have shown promise in persons who have a small focal defect (full thickness cartilage loss with an area less than 2 square cm) - the majority of people with symptomatic osteoarthritis typically have widespread damage through the joint making this procedure more technically difficult and the results less favourable. There is no point in undergoing an experimental surgical procedure if the chances of success (marked improvement in symptoms) are negligible. There is currently a great deal of research being conducted in these and other tissue-engineering techniques that may prove effective long term. Until they do (in the absence of being involved in a research study) please resist the temptation of having this therapy.

Other surgical options

There are several other techniques that are occasionally offered to people with arthritis. One such procedure is microfracture. This operation, which is performed by keyhole surgery, entails making holes in the bone surfaces with a drill or pick to encourage new cartilage to grow. The benefits are not well proven and the results are not as good as knee replacement for advanced arthritis.

Arthroplasty/joint replacement

Surgery may be used to replace a damaged joint with an artificial joint. Development of modern total hip arthroplasty in the 1960s by John Charnley, a British surgeon, represents a milestone in orthopaedic surgery.

Joint replacement is an irreversible intervention used in those for whom other treatment modalities have failed. Arthroplasty, or joint replacement surgery, is most often done to repair hips and knees, but also is used to repair shoulders, elbows, fingers, ankles and toes. Currently the most common indication for knee (total knee replacement or TKR) and hip replacement (THR) (approximately 85 per cent of all cases) is osteoarthritis. Each year, approximately 300,000 TKR surgeries are performed in the USA for end-stage arthritis of the knee joint. Over 30,000 knee replacement operations are carried out each year in England and Wales, and the number is increasing.

Who should have their joint replaced?

To be a candidate for joint replacement you should have radiographic evidence of joint damage, moderate to severe persistent pain that is not adequately relieved by an extended course of non-surgical management, and clinically significant functional limitation resulting in diminished quality of life (Mancuso et al. 1996). Joint replacement surgery dramatically relieves pain in people with severe osteoarthritis of the hip or knee, and this benefit appears to last for at least three years. However, it may take up to one year before the benefits of joint replacement surgery become fully apparent.

Joint replacement is an elective procedure, and the risks and outcomes vary. Therefore, it is essential that you be informed of the likely consequences of the surgery in terms that are specific to you. Everyone's goals and expectations (i.e. hopes and fears) should be considered before surgery to determine whether these goals are attainable and the expectations realistic. Any discrepancies between your expectations and the likely surgical outcome should be discussed in detail with the surgeon before surgery.

There are few absolute contraindications for joint replacement other than active local (where the joint is replaced) or systemic infection (infection elsewhere such as urinary tract infection or pneumonia) and other medical conditions that can substantially increase the risk of serious operative complications or death. Obesity is not a contraindication to joint replacement; however, there may be an increased risk of delayed wound healing and perioperative infection in obese patients. Severe peripheral vascular disease and some neurologic impairments are both relative contraindications to joint replacement.

With proper patient selection, good to excellent results can be expected in 95 per cent of patients, and the survival rate of the implant is expected to be 95 per cent at 15 years (Callahan et al. 1994). When overall health improvement is used to assess the cost-effectiveness of total joint arthroplasty, the hip and knee arthroplasty have similar results (Ethgen et al. 2004). Costs associated with long-term medication, assistive care and decreased work productivity may exceed the cost of arthroplasty (Segal et al. 2004).

It should be noted that joint replacement is more cost-effective among patients who had the most to gain (those with lower preoperative function). However, if left until functional status has declined, the postoperative functional status does not improve to the level achieved by those with higher preoperative function (Fortin *et al.* 1999). Please don't defer the surgery until your function is too impaired; for example if you are wheelchair or bed-bound for a long time before the surgery your postoperative recovery will be very difficult and prolonged.

What happens during joint replacement?

During joint replacement surgery, the surgeon first removes all the damaged bone and cartilage from the joint. Surgeons may replace affected joints with artificial joints called prostheses. These joints can be made from metal alloys, high-density plastic and ceramic material. Surgeons choose the design and components of prostheses according to their patient's weight, sex, age, activity level and other medical conditions. They can be joined to bone surfaces by special cements. Artificial joints can wear out and about 10 per cent of artificial joints may need replacing again.

For younger people who are more active or for older people who have strong bones, doctors sometimes use artificial joints that do not require cement to stay in place. These artificial joints are designed with spaces into which the

Before   After

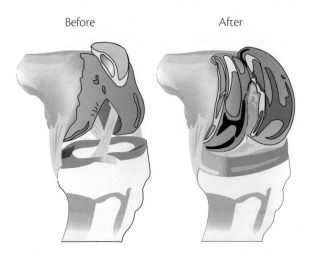

Figure 17.4 A prosthesis is a device designed to replace a missing part of the body, or to make a part of the body work better. The metal prosthetic device in knee-joint replacement surgery replaces cartilage and bone that is damaged from disease or ageing.

person's own bone can grow, holding the artificial joint in place more naturally. By avoiding the use of cement, which can weaken over time, these types of artificial joints usually stay in place longer than those that are held in place with cement. In patients younger than age 55, alternative surgical procedures, such as osteotomy and unicompartmental knee replacement, deserve consideration.

Recovery from joint replacement surgery depends on several factors, including a person's general health and level of activity before the surgery. For this reason, it is not a good idea to put off the surgery for long. The more active you are before your surgery, the faster your recovery is likely to be. Most people who have a hip or knee replaced will need physical therapy to help regain their mobility. A physical therapist will recommend special exercises to help you build up the muscles around your new artificial joint. Physical therapy starts in the hospital shortly after surgery and continues after you are home.

What complications can arise?

A replacement joint can never be as good as a natural joint. You are still likely to experience some difficulties in movement. Although complications from joint replacement are rare, the new joint can become infected or slip out of place. For this reason, your doctor will ask you to come in regularly for check-ups so that they can monitor your healing and recovery.

Any operation on the lower limbs can lead to a small blood clot forming in the leg. To reduce the risk of blood clots, your doctor may prescribe anti-clotting medication. If a clot develops it is usually treated with blood-thinning medicines such as heparin or warfarin. In a very small number of cases the blood clot can travel to the lungs (pulmonary embolism), which leads to breathlessness and chest pains.

Joint replacement surgery may also cause bleeding and infection in the period just after surgery. The use of pre-operative antibiotics and other operating room procedures reduces the risk of deep wound infections after replacement surgery to less than 1 per cent.

Loosening of the attachment between the hardware and bones may also occur and require removal and replacement of the artificial joint. Debris caused by wear of the plastic or metal sometimes causes inflammation and may also require reoperation to correct if the replacement becomes loose.

Removing and replacing an artificial joint is more difficult than the initial surgery and has a higher risk of complications, especially of infection. Because of the limited life of artificial joints, people with osteoarthritis are generally encouraged to wait as long as possible before having replacement surgery. Age younger than 55 at the time of replacement surgery, male gender, obesity, and presence of comorbid conditions are all risk factors for revision.

Proper surgical technique, surgeon's experience and the choice of prosthesis (device designed to replace part of the body) may have important influences on surgical outcomes. One of the clearest associations with better outcomes appears to be the higher procedure volume of the individual surgeon and the procedure volume of the hospital. Overall the risk of death, usually due to a heart attack, a stroke, or a blood clot reaching the lungs, is about 1 in 200 (0.5 per cent), but this risk varies between patients and hospitals.

What are the options for joint replacements?

Total knee replacement

Most joint replacement operations involve a total joint replacement which means that both sides (compartments) of the joint are replaced.

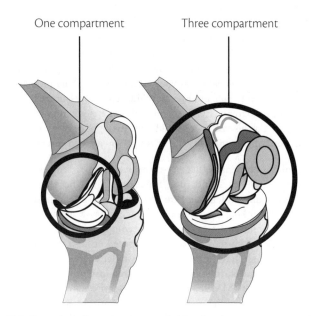

One compartment   Three compartment

Figure 17.5 Figure depicting unicompartmental (one) replacement versus total knee replacement – replacement of both tibiofemoral and patellofemoral (kneecap) compartments.

Unicompartmental replacement

If arthritis affects only one side of your knee – usually the inner side – it may be possible to have a half-knee or unicompartmental replacement (sometimes called hemiarthroplasty). The unicompartmental operation is only suitable for about 1 in 4 people with osteoarthritis. This is a less extensive operation than a total knee replacement and it should therefore mean a quicker recovery.

Kneecap replacement

It is possible to replace just the kneecap (patella) and its groove (trochlea) if this is the only part of your knee which is affected by arthritis. This is also called a patellofemoral replacement or patellofemoral joint arthroplasty. Again this is a less major operation with speedier recovery times. The operation is only really suitable for about 1 in 10 people with osteoarthritis.

What happens in hospital?

Pre-operative visit

If you and your doctors agree you should go ahead with a knee replacement operation you will usually be invited to a pre-operative assessment clinic some time before your planned admission date. At this visit you will be assessed by a doctor or nurse to see if you are generally fit enough to cope with the operation. This will involve a number of tests. Usually samples of blood are taken to check that you are not anaemic and that your kidneys are working properly. A urine sample will be taken to rule out infection. Your blood pressure will be recorded and an electrocardiograph (ECG) tracing will be carried out to make sure your heart is healthy. At this visit you should have the opportunity to ask any questions about your operation or discuss anything you are concerned about.

There is general consensus that pre-operative heart-risk assessment should be performed and heart and lung function should be optimized before TKR. If there is any underlying heart or lung disease this should be treated preoperatively. Smoking cessation can reduce the risk of cardiac events and postoperative pneumonia and should be recommended for all smokers pre-operatively, although it may need to be initiated at least two months before surgery for optimal effect. Among patients older than age 70, preoperative assessment of mental status with a standardized instrument such as the Mini Mental Status Exam (MMSE) can help to identify patients at high risk for confusion at the time of the operation. Postoperatively, incentive spirometry (breathing exercises) should be used to reduce the incidence of pneumonia. Pre-operative patient education about what will happen during surgery and the postoperative period has been shown to improve patient outcomes, including reduced use of pain medications, reduced anxiety, and improved patient satisfaction.

Going into hospital

You will probably be admitted to hospital on the day of your operation or the evening before. You will be asked to sign a form consenting to surgery, and your joint will be marked for the operation.

Anaesthesia

The operation will be performed under a general or spinal anaesthetic so that you feel no pain.

The operation

This usually takes between 45 minutes and 2 hours, depending on the complexity of the surgery.

After the operation

Before going back to the ward you will spend some time in the recovery room. Here you may be given more fluids and drugs, such as painkillers, through the tube in your arm. You may be given a switch so that you can administer painkillers to yourself at a safe rate according to how much pain you feel. Oxygen therapy is likely to be given through a mask or through tubes into your nose. If necessary you will be given a blood transfusion.

Getting mobile again

After the first day or so, the various tubes giving painkillers, fluids or oxygen therapy will be removed and, with the help of nursing staff and physiotherapists, you should be able to start walking. The length of time it will take you to become mobile will vary according to your circumstances and the outcome of your operation.

Generally, if you have had a spinal anaesthetic or nerve block you will have very little feeling in your leg for the first day or two. You may have a tube (catheter) inserted into your bladder for a few days to help you pass water, especially if both knees have been replaced at the same time.

At first you will need crutches or a frame to walk. Your physiotherapist will be able to advise you on climbing stairs and other activities and should also explain the exercises you will need to do in order to keep improving your mobility in hospital and at home.

Going home

It is usually possible to go home as soon as your wound is healing well and you can safely walk to and from the toilet, get dressed, and manage stairs with the help of crutches or a frame. Most people are fit to go home between 4 and 9 days after surgery, but it may be longer in some cases.

Before you leave hospital do ask your occupational therapist or physiotherapist about the best ways to get dressed, take a bath, get in and out of bed, and use the toilet, and about any dressing or bathing aids that you may need. This is especially important if you have had both knees replaced at the same time.

Follow-up appointments

You will usually have a follow-up hospital appointment about six weeks after your operation to check on your recovery.

When will I get back to normal?

Obviously it will be some weeks before you recover from your operation and start to feel the benefits of your new knee/hip joint. You can make a big difference to how quickly you become mobile again by making sure you follow the advice of your hospital team and keeping up your exercises. You should make sure you have no major commitments – including long-haul air travel – for the first six weeks after the operation.

Gradually you will be able to build up the exercises to strengthen your muscles so that you can move more easily and independently. You will probably need painkillers as the exercises can be painful at first. Your physiotherapist or occupational therapist should advise you on these tasks but here are a few pointers:

- **Walking.** It is important at first that you do not twist your knee/hip as you turn around. Take small steps instead. It should be possible to walk outside about three weeks after your surgery but make sure you wear good supportive outdoor shoes.

- **Going up and down stairs.** When going up the stairs use the handrail and hold your crutch or crutches in your free hand. First put your unoperated leg onto the step, place your crutches on the stair with your free hand, then move your operated leg up. When you go down the stairs, it is the other way round. Put your operated leg down first with your crutches, followed by your unoperated leg.

- **Sitting.** Make sure you do not sit with your legs crossed for the first six weeks.

- **Sleeping.** You do not have to sleep in a special position after knee surgery, as you would after a hip replacement. However, you should avoid lying with a pillow underneath your knee. Although this may feel comfortable it can result in a permanently bent knee.

- **Driving.** If you were driving before your operation, you should be able to drive again after about six weeks if your knee replacement was carried out by the conventional method, or about three weeks if you had minimally invasive surgery.

References

Brouwer, R. W., Jakma, T. S., Bierma-Zeinstra, S. M., Verhagen, A. P., Verhaar, J. (2005) *Osteotomy for treating knee osteoarthritis.* [Review] [36 refs]. *Cochrane Database of Systematic Reviews* (1): CD004019.

Callahan, C. M., Drake, B. G., Heck, D. A., Dittus, R. S. (1994) Patient outcomes following tricompartmental total knee replacement. A meta-analysis. *JAMA* 271(17): 1349–1357.

Ethgen, O., Bruyere, O., Richy, F., Dardennes, C., Reginster, J. Y. (2004) Health-related quality of life in total hip and total knee arthroplasty. A qualitative and systematic review of the literature. [Review] [150 refs]. *Journal of Bone and Joint Surgery – American* 86-A(5): 963–974.

Fortin, P. R., Clarke, A. E., Joseph, L., Liang, M. H., Tanzer, M., Ferland, D. *et al.* (1999) Outcomes of total hip and knee replacement: preoperative functional status predicts outcomes at six months after surgery. *Arthritis and Rheumatism* 42(8): 1722–1728.

Mancuso, C. A., Ranawat, C. S., Esdaile, J. M., Johanson, N. A., Charlson, M. E. (1996) Indications for total hip and total knee arthroplasties. Results of orthopaedic surveys. *Journal of Arthroplasty* 11(1): 34–46.

Moseley, J. B., O'Malley, K., Petersen, N. J., Menke, T. J., Brody, B. A., Kuykendall, D. H. *et al.* (2002) A controlled trial of arthroscopic surgery for osteoarthritis of the knee.[Comment][Summary for patients in *J Fam Pract* 2002 Oct; 51(10):813; PMID: 12401143]. *New England Journal of Medicine* 347(2): 81–88.

Naudie, D., Bourne, R. B., Rorabeck, C. H., Bourne, T. J. (1999) The Install Award. Survivorship of the high tibial valgus osteotomy. A 10- to -22-year follow-up study. *Clinical Orthopaedics and Related Research* (367): 18–27.

Segal, L., Day, S. E., Chapman, A. B., Osborne, R. H. (2004) Can we reduce disease burden from osteoarthritis? [Comment]. *Medical Journal of Australia* 180(5 Suppl): S11–S17.

Stukenborg-Colsman, C., Wirth, C. J., Lazovic, D., Wefer, A. (2001) High tibial osteotomy versus unicompartmental joint replacement in unicompartmental knee joint osteoarthritis: 7–10-year follow-up prospective randomised study. *Knee* 8(3): 187–194.

18

Complementary therapies

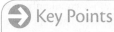 Key Points

⬥ Complementary therapies can play an important role in encouraging positive changes in lifestyle and outlook, such as increased self-reliance, a positive attitude, relaxation practices and appropriate exercises.

⬥ Lifestyle changes like these may help to improve the pain and other symptoms stemming from osteoarthritis.

⬥ When choosing a complementary therapy please use your common sense and be properly informed.

Complementary therapies for osteoarthritis have become more popular and more widely available to the general public. According to recent surveys in many Western countries nearly half of all persons with OA are trying some kind of unconventional therapy. This trend to complementary medicine suggests that patients are increasingly dissatisfied with conventional medicine and/or concerned about the side-effects of prescribed medications.

In general, conventional medical treatments are safe and effective, but more often than not drugs and surgery cannot fully control the symptoms of OA. Thus it is not surprising that one of the most common complaints taken to complementary practitioners is the persistent pain and limited function that occurs with OA, despite these more conventional treatments. With no known cure it is often expected that this persistent discomfort or limited function has to be endured. It may be as a consequence of this that many persons affected with OA then seek out complementary therapies.

What are complementary therapies?

There are a wide variety of complementary therapies that range from ancient systems of medicine such as homoeopathy and herbalism, to treatments such as massage and aromatherapy. A therapy is considered complementary or alternative if it's not traditionally been used in conventional medicine—but this is changing.

Until well into the twentieth century, many of the therapies we now call complementary were mainstream medicine. Doctors prescribed herbs and other plant-based medicines, and did massage and manipulations. Mental attitudes, such as faith and the will to live, were considered an important part of healing, and prevention was a major form of healthcare. Many of these therapies are still considered mainstream medicine in other cultures.

Meanwhile, advances in medical science led to a more technical (potentially less person-friendly), intervention-based healthcare that we commonly refer to as Western medicine. The results of this type of care have been spectacular. Vaccines protect us from a range of deadly diseases, antibiotics are truly life-saving and surgery can perform wonders. Our lifespan has been extended from an average age of 48 at the beginning of the twentieth century to 76 as we entered the new millennium. With these advances in medical technology, most medical schools stopped teaching the older, more time-consuming treatments. In addition medical practices developed concern for their own fiscal responsibilities and constrained the length of visits and thus patient–doctor interaction and encouraged procedures that generate more income. In this less than patient-friendly environment it is not surprising that people affected by chronic diseases seek help elsewhere.

Often people want to turn back the clock by returning to complementary medicine. Part of it is the frustration with today's impersonal healthcare system but equally important is the disappointment that, despite a wealth of medical research, cures have still not been discovered for chronic illnesses such as OA. Although Western medicine excels at treating acute ills such as infections, emergencies and accidents, there are still relatively few treatments for illnesses that drag out over years or even decades. We are living longer with chronic diseases that are more complex to treat. They usually have more than one cause, and no simple solutions.

Alternative therapies may offer tools and remedies that, along with mainstream medicine, can influence your overall health. For example, there is evidence that emotions and mental attitudes can have a major impact in the long-term management of chronic illness. An interest in alternative therapies shows that you want to take a more active role in your healthcare, and the sense of control that you gain by becoming involved in managing your OA can contribute to your overall well-being.

Choosing a complementary therapy

There are two important principles to follow when considering using a complementary therapy: be properly informed and use your common sense. There's no free lunch, and there are no miracle cures for OA.

Unconventional therapies are remedies that, along with mainstream medicine, may improve your symptoms—and may not. Weigh the risks and benefits as well as the costs in time and money, and know when to quit a therapy that isn't working for you. Ask your doctor to be your partner as you explore adding unconventional therapies to your treatment plan. Assuming you have a good working relationship with your doctor and that your communication is not hindered by paternalistic, conservative attitudes, it is much safer to communicate your thoughts about seeking out alternative therapies with your doctor.

Do not expect a cure from complementary therapies—irrespective of what you may be told by some alternative health practitioners. What you can hope for with some of these therapies is that you gain more control over your symptoms and hopefully as a result regain more control over how they affect your life. When used in combination with conventional medicines, they may help you feel better and live a fuller life.

Before you commit to a complementary therapy, a few words of caution. The basic principle of conventional treatment that all doctors observe is that you do not harm the patient. Before you decide to try a complementary therapy, here are some common sense suggestions to help you avoid inadvertently harming yourself.

- *Get an accurate diagnosis:* make sure you know from your doctor specifically what type of arthritis or musculo-skeletal disorder you have, so you know what you're treating.

- *Consult with your doctor:* seek your doctor's advice about the complementary therapy you are considering and whether there will be any interaction between the therapy and the medications or other treatments you're taking. Always tell your doctor everything you are taking or doing, including over the counter drugs, herbs, vitamins and special diets or exercises.

- *Check the therapist's qualifications:* if the therapy is regulated, check whether the therapist or practitioner has a licence or certificate, or whether they are certified by a professional organization. Find out what sort of training they have done and where it was done.

◆ *Consider the time and cost:* find out details about costs and how many treatments you'll need to see some effect. Check whether your health insurance covers this therapy—arrangements vary between insurers and standard health cover usually doesn't include complementary treatments.

Be aware of these danger signs

Some types of complementary therapies are regulated and many practitioners have high standards of professional ethics and practice. However, others are not regulated—and unfortunately, not all practitioners are ethical or competent.

Be suspicious of any health professional who does the following:

1. Promises you can be 'cured'. Many therapies may help your OA, but there is no cure.

2. Tells you to stop or decrease prescription medicines. Never stop or change doses of prescription medicines without talking to your doctor.

3. Advises a severely restricted diet. This doesn't mean a vegetarian diet but a diet that is extreme or involves eliminating many types of foods. If you want to go this route, ask your doctor for a referral to a nutritionally oriented doctor or to a registered dietitian who will help you plan a well-balanced diet.

4. Insists you pay in advance for a series of expensive treatments. No practitioner can predict how you might respond to a treatment, and you should not have to pay for treatments you do not receive or need.

5. Cannot show you a licence or a certificate from an approved school or organisation in his or her specialty. Anyone can claim to be an expert—ask for proof!

6. Advises you to keep the treatment a secret from your doctor, or anyone else. Good medical treatments are not secrets—they are shared in the medical community. Your doctor and your spouse or partner (or at least one member of your family or a good friend) should know the details of your medical treatment, in case of emergency.

What are the main differences between conventional medicine and complementary therapies?

While the different types of complementary therapies have very different philosophies and practices, most share a common view of health and healing: they emphasize 'wellness', which they believe comes from a balance between the body, the mind and the environment. Illness happens when there is an 'imbalance' between these factors.

Conventional (allopathic) medicine tries to treat the specific part of the body which is 'faulty', whereas complementary therapies concentrate on the whole person—the so-called holistic approach. Each person is treated as a unique individual who has their own inner resources to fight and overcome illness.

Conventional treatment encourages the patient to remain relatively passive and to accept their diagnosis and treatment. Complementary therapies demand that you actively participate in your treatment. The holistic approach of complementary therapies means you usually have to make more lifestyle changes (that is, changes to your diet, exercise and mental attitude) than conventional treatments. This may be key to their continuing success with those who have tried them.

Both conventional treatments and complementary therapies emphasize the quality of the relationship between the practitioner and the patient. A good (open and communicative) relationship is essential for a successful outcome.

How do complementary therapies work?

We all know that the body heals itself, that cuts and wounds heal and that the body's cells are routinely replaced. Complementary therapists believe that this self-healing is the basis of all healing. Complementary therapy aims to help the individual get well and then stay healthy. The basic idea is that people 'heal themselves' with the help of a trained practitioner.

What complementary therapies are there?

The main complementary therapies that are used in OA appear in alphabetical order below.

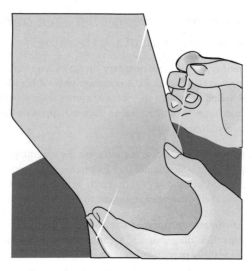

Figure 18.1 Placement of fine needles at precise points in the knee has demonstrated efficacy in pain relief.

Acupuncture

Acupuncture uses fine needles inserted at precise points on the body. It's been used for centuries (originated in China more than 2000 years ago) in Chinese medicine to restore health for a variety of conditions. Traditional Chinese acupuncture is based on the theory that illness can result when the body's flow of energy (called *chi* or *qi*) is blocked or imbalanced. The acupuncture needles are positioned to correct those problems. Western medical practitioners have become interested in acupuncture, especially for pain relief. However, they often view acupuncture differently from their peers in traditional Chinese medicine, focusing on its biochemical effects instead of energy flow. In 2002, acupuncture was used by an estimated 2.1 million adults in the USA, according to the Centers for Disease Control and Prevention's 2002 National Health Interview Survey. The acupuncture technique that has been most studied scientifically involves penetrating the skin with thin, solid, metallic needles that are manipulated by the hands or by electrical stimulation. Recently a number of well-controlled studies have examined the efficacy of acupuncture for pain relief in knee OA. In general these have been supportive of a moderate effect with most patients demonstrating a 40 per cent decrease in pain, and a nearly 40 per cent improvement in knee function. This may prove to be a very useful adjunct to other therapies and probably much less damaging than some therapies such as non-steroidal anti-inflammatories.

Aromatherapy

Plant extracts have been used for health and well-being for many centuries. In aromatherapy, the essential oils are inhaled, massaged into the skin or used in a bath. How these oils work is not entirely understood. Some therapists believe that the essential oil is the 'soul' of the plant which has powerful properties to uplift your spirit as well as help with more fundamental health problems.

Each essential oil is made up of chemical components which are believed to have individual therapeutic properties but some of these chemicals can be poisonous (toxic) in large quantities or can harm people with certain conditions such as pregnancy or epilepsy. This is why professional aromatherapists have to understand the chemical components of each oil.

Copper bangles

Many people with OA wear copper bangles. Research has shown that people with OA do have enough copper in their bodies for normal health, so it is difficult to understand what effect these bangles can have. There is no research supporting the use of copper bangles.

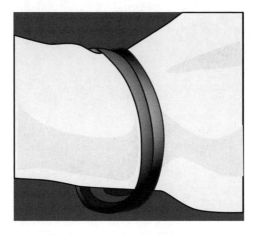

Figure 18.2 Copper bangle.

Dietary supplements

Coral calcium

Coral calcium is usually bought in sachets and drunk sprinkled in water. One company that sells this claims that the residents of the Japanese islands where it is collected live very long and healthy lives because of the natural elements in the water, such as calcium, magnesium and other minerals. Suppliers claim that tiny particles of coral release these elements when put in water and that these elements then help the body's auto-immune system. There has been no serious research so far into the effectiveness and safety of coral calcium.

Green-lipped mussel extract

Green-lipped mussel extract comes from New Zealand. As with many conventional medicines, several studies found it helpful while other studies showed no helpful effect. It appears to do no harm, but we do not really know whether it can help your OA.

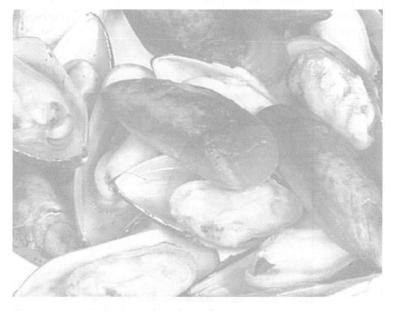

Figure 18.3 New Zealand green-lipped mussels.

Herbal medicine

Herbal medicine has been present throughout history. Today about one-quarter of pharmaceutical preparations contain at least one active ingredient extracted from plant sources. Whereas conventional medicine tries to isolate the active ingredient of a plant, herbal remedies use the whole plant. Herbalists argue that the natural chemical balance in the whole plant has a better effect on the body than giving a patient just the active ingredient. Herbal treatment uses plants to try to mobilize the self-healing powers of the body.

Herbal remedies are very popular with some people who believe that they help to cure different forms of arthritis. Some clinical trials have found some benefits, but there is not yet enough information about any specific herb to be absolutely certain about their effects.

If herbal remedies are going to work, you usually need to take them for about three months before you feel the full benefit. They are usually safe (non-toxic) but they may sometimes, like drugs, cause side-effects. These side-effects can include nervous depression, irritability, sleeplessness, and even aches and pains in the muscles or joints. If you are thinking of using these remedies, make sure you buy them from a reputable manufacturer to ensure product quality.

Homeopathy

Homeopathy is a 200-year-old system of medicine. It is based upon the Law of Similars (let like be cured by like—so a treatment for nausea might be a substance that can make you feel sick). The effectiveness of homeopathic medicines or remedies depends on how they are made. The original, wholly natural substance is diluted many times in water or alcohol so that only a few molecules of the original substance may survive in the final remedy. An important part of this process is agitation of the liquid between dilutions—this process is thought to maintain the potency of the original substance.

You can easily buy homeopathic remedies over the counter in health food shops and pharmacies. Homeopathy usually also requires a change in lifestyle to complement the treatment, which could include changing your diet, more relaxation or exercise. Medically qualified homeopaths can also use orthodox medicine if they wish, as well as the medicines they use in homeopathy. They can prescribe homeopathy in a truly complementary manner.

Most doctors find that if a chemical drug provides benefits then it can also do harm if it is wrongly applied or given in the wrong dosage. This rarely happens with homeopathic preparations. A number of carefully controlled trials have been carried out with homeopathic medicine, some of them involving arthritis. These suggest that homeopathy can help, but we cannot say if a specific remedy 'works' for hay fever or arthritis. Homeopathic remedies need to be prescribed on an individual basis, so there is no particular remedy for OA, rather they are prescribed for the individual who may have OA.

Magnetic therapy

It has been suggested that certain types of magnetic fields can help speed up healing and reduce pain in muscular complaints. Physiotherapists use equipment which produces a pulsed magnetic field for this purpose. You may also have seen products such as magnetic bracelets advertised. The manufacturers of these claim that the magnetic field can increase the ability of the blood to carry oxygen and waste products and that people with osteoarthritis and other conditions have reported benefits. However, the bracelets should not be worn by anyone who has a heart pacemaker fitted. Evidence on whether magnetism applied in this way can help osteoarthritis is not conclusive at the moment.

Massage

Massage has been around for thousands of years, and was probably first used in China. Massage can be stimulating or sedating, vigorous or gentle, and include the whole body or only parts of it. Oils, creams, lotions or even talcum powder are used. Massage can reduce your anxiety and stress levels, relieve muscular tension and fatigue, improve circulation and thus reduce pain levels. It is generally very safe and relaxing, and a trained massage therapist will typically follow strict guidelines to avoid endangering patients.

Osteopathy

Osteopathy is a system of manual medicine where the hands are used to diagnose and treat a patient. There are no harmful side-effects, and osteopaths are taught to use minimal force. It was developed in the late nineteenth century by an American doctor, who saw the body as a finely tuned, fully integrated machine, not as a collection of parts.

Osteopaths believe that a problem with the mechanical structure of the body will impair its function, but that the body will heal itself if it is given the right circumstances; that is, a balanced and healthy lifestyle, or the help of osteopathic manipulation. Ailments such as headaches, skin disorders and digestive disorders are seen as the results of spinal misalignment. Osteopaths believe that their manipulation of the muscles and joints helps the body to combat illness and heal itself.

Reflexology

Reflexology is a treatment in which varying degrees of pressure are applied to different parts of the body to promote health and well-being. It suggests that every part of the body is connected by reflex zones or pathways which terminate in the soles of the feet, palms of the hands, ears, tongue and head.

Reflexology suggests that tension, congestion or some other imbalance will affect an entire zone and that it is possible to treat one part of the zone to change another part of the body. Gentle pressure is thought to help detoxification and promote healing. It can be very relaxing, and thus diminish pain, but there is no evidence to suggest it can directly affect your OA.

Complementary therapies can play an important role in encouraging positive changes in lifestyle and outlook, such as increased self-reliance, a positive attitude, relaxation practices and appropriate exercises. Lifestyle changes like these may help to improve the pain and other symptoms stemming from OA. Currently a cure for OA is not possible, and these changes can be as important as more conventional treatments.

Useful addresses

National Institute of Arthritis and Musculoskeletal and Skin Diseases: http://www.niams.nih.gov

Arthritis Foundation (US): http://www.arthritis.org

Arthritis Research Campaign (UK): http://www.arc.org.uk

American College of Rheumatology: http://www.rheumatology.org

Johns Hopkins Arthritis Centre Website: http://www.hopkins-arthritis.som.jhmi.edu/rheumatoid/rheum.html

Diagnostic and Therapeutic Guidelines: http://www.hopkins-arthritis.som.jhmi.edu/acr/class_rheum

Support groups

Arthritis Care (UK)

Arthritis Care is the UK's largest organization, working with all people who have arthritis to provide information and support. They are a user-led organization meaning that people with arthritis are integrally involved in all of their activities.

Tel: 0808 800 4050

Website: http://www.arthritiscare.org.uk.

Arthritis Foundation (US)

The Arthritis Foundation in the US is the only national not-for-profit organization that supports the more than 100 types of arthritis and related conditions with advocacy, programmes, services and research. General queries for arthritis-related information and materials:

Tel: 404 872 7100 or 1 800 568 4045

Website: http://www.arthritis.org

Arthritis Research Campaign (ARC)

Website: http://www.arc.org.uk

Diet and arthritis

Website: http://www.arthritis.org/resources/Nutrition/diet.asp

Website: http://www.arc.org.uk/arthinfo/patpubs/6010/6010.asp

Exercise and arthritis

Website: http://www.niams.nih.gov/hi/topics/arthritis/arthexfs.htm

Website: http://www.arthritis.org/conditions/exercise/default.asp

http://www.hopkins-arthritis.som.jhmi.edu/mngmnt/exercise.html

Hydrotherapy

Website: http://www.arc.org.uk/about_arth/infosheets/6254/6254.htm

Growing Stronger: Strength Training for Older Adults

Website: http://www.nutrition.tufts.edu/research/growingstronger

NIAMS information on joint replacement surgery

http://www.niams.nih.gov/hi/topics/arthritis/jointrep.htm

NIH Consensus Development Conference on Total Knee Replacement

Website: http://consensus.nih.gov/2003/2003TotalKneeReplacement117html.htm

Questions and answers about hip replacement

Website: http://www.niams.nih.gov/hi/topics/hip/hiprepqa.htm

T'ai chi

See the publication *Overcoming Arthritis* (Dorling Kindersley Publishers 2002) by Dr Paul Lam and Judith Horstman, which contains 160 photos with detailed instructions and information about T'ai chi and arthritis.

Website: http://www.taichiproductions.com

Yoga

For more information about yoga, see the website of the International Association of Yoga Therapists.

Website: http://www.iayt.org

For some poses see http://www.abc-of-yoga.com/yoga-and-health/yoga-for-arthritis.asp

Glossary

Abduction: of a joint means to move it away from the midline of the body, e.g. standing straight and lifting one foot off the ground and moving it outwards.

Acetabular dysplasia: the cup-like shape of the hip bone is slightly abnormal in shape so as not to securely support the femur and often necessitates surgery.

Acupuncture: this originated in China over 2000 years ago and is based on the foundation that good health relies on an equal balance of forces that then ensure a good body flow of energy – *chi* or *qi*. It believes that ill health is the response to an imbalance of these forces. Acupuncture needles are inserted over certain pathways with the aim of stimulating the brain to release chemicals that can improve general well-being and promote healing. In more recent times the Western world has developed acupuncture using a more biological approach to promote general well-being.

Analgesia: means pain relief.

Ambulatory devices: are aids that can help you with walking such as crutches, walking sticks, and frames.

Ambulatory pain: pain experienced when walking.

Analgesics: this is the name given to drugs that relieve pain, e.g. paracetemol, NSAIDs, mild opioids, strong opioids.

Aromatherapy: this is the use of plant extracts to help health and well-being. It is used in the form of massage oils, inhaled, or used in baths.

Arthrocentesis: the puncture and aspiration of a joint.

Arthrodesis: a form of surgery that fuses joints together and in so doing immobilizes the joint.

Arthroplasty: a form of surgery that changes the joint, for instance a joint replacement.

Arthroscopic debridement: a form of surgery that involves inserting a narrow tube into the joint through which instruments are passed to enable the surgeon to take out flaky pieces of cartilage, or loose pieces of bone.

Arthroscopy: a form of surgery that involves inserting a narrowing tube into the joint through which the surgeon can conduct an examination (and also perform some surgical procedures).

Articular capsule: is the name given to two layers of connective tissue that surround the structures of the joint.

Body mass index *also called the BMI*: it is the standard scientific table used in medicine to ascertain the desirable weight we should strive to maintain for good health. It is calculated by dividing the weight in kg by the height in m^2. We should be aiming for 25 or less.

Bouchard's nodes: these are the bony nodules found on the proximal phalangeal joint (joint between the knuckle and small joint at the end of each finger).

Capital femoral epiphysis: slipped capital femoral epiphysis (SCFE) is a hip problem that starts if the epiphysis (growing end) of the femur (thigh bone) slips from the ball of the hip joint.

Cartilage: is found at the end of the bones and stops the bones rubbing together and also acts as a shock absorber.

Chondrocytes: cells that make cartilage.

Chondroitin: a naturally occurring substance found in the cartilage that is part of the protein that gives cartilage its elasticity.

Collagen: fibres found within the cartilage that give it its structure and strength.

Complementary therapies: the umbrella name given to a host of therapies that are not considered part of conventional medicine, e.g. acupuncture, aromatherapy, reflexology, herbal medicine, and homeopathy.

Congentital: a condition you are born with.

Contralateral: the opposite side.

Corticosteroids: these are hormones that are either produced naturally or synthetically. They have various metabolic functions and are able to reduce inflammation.

Crepitus: a crunching felt on moving the joint.

Cruciate ligaments: the ligaments found in the knee joint.

Cysts: an abnormal sac in the bone near the joint containing a liquid substance.

Degenerative joint disease: is another term for OA, it means the deterioration of the joint over time.

Distal: farthest away, for instance the distal phalangeal joint is the finger joint farthest from the body.

Effusion: fluid within the joint.

Endochondral ossification: the formation of bone tissue within cartilage; the process by which bones grow in length. Local risk factors of osteoarthritis are factors that are specific to a joint such as meniscal damage in the knee or muscle weakness around the joint.

Endorphins: naturally occurring chemicals in the body that create analgesia and a sense of well-being.

Erthyrocyte sedimentation rate: a blood test that establishes inflammation within the body.

Essential fatty acids (EFA): these are fats that the body can not produce for itself, they are obtained by eating foods that contain them. The body uses them to make chemicals (prostaglandins and leukotrienes) that can reduce the breakdown of cartilage and reduce inflammation.

Gait: is the term given to ones natural walking technique, some clinicians may describe it as unsteady (as risk of falling) or wide (steps are taken in a wide fashion).

Glucosamine: naturally occurring component of the cartilage, also found in shellfish and synthetically manufactured. It is now widely used in the field of OA as it can reduce pain and also help remodel cartilage.

Gout: a form of arthritis associated with an excess of uric acid in the body.

Heberden's nodes: nodes found on the distal phalangeal joint in severe hand OA.

Homeopathy: a 200-year-old form of medicine based in treating like on like to cure (for instance if you wish to be cured of your sickness then the treatment would be to cause the sickness). Small quantities of a substance are diluted down so that only a few molecules are present and then they are administered.

Hyaline cartilage: the cartilage that is affected in osteoarthritis, it is found in most moving joints.

Hyaluronic acid: a naturally occurring component of the synovial fluid and found in the cartilage. In OA there is a depletion of this and hence an intra-articular injection of hyaluronic acid may be indicated.

Hydrotherapy: a form of physiotherapy that is conducted in water.

Intra-articular injections: injections that are passed directly into the joint.

Lateral: on the outside.

Ligaments: these are strong fibrous tissues that connect bone to bone and in so doing play a role in keeping the joint secure and stable.

Local risk factors of osteoarthritis: are factors that are specific to osteoarthritis.

Medial: on the inside.

Menisci: these are found within the knee joint and are little spacers, that is they help pad out the knee joint to prevent structures collapsing on each other. Some people refer to these as cartilage but that is incorrect.

Micronutrients: necessary chemicals often in minute amounts that are required by our body for normal growth and development.

Mild opioids: these are the milder forms of opioids and are chemical substances that have a morphine-like action in the body.

Mitochondria: a structure in the cytoplasm of all cells except bacteria in which food molecules (sugars, fatty acids, and amino acids) are broken down in the presence of oxygen and converted to energy.

Neutraceutical: a food or naturally occurring food supplement thought to have a beneficial effect on human health.

NSAID: non-steroidal anti-inflammatory drugs.

Opioids: an opioid is a chemical substance that has a morphine-like action in the body.

Osteopathy: osteopathy is a non-invasive manual medicine that focuses on total body health by treating and strengthening the musculoskeletal framework, which includes the joints, muscles, and spine.

Osteophytes: osteophytes are bone and cartilage that forms in a joint with osteoarthritis. Osteophytes can develop as marginal (on the periphery of joints) or central (mostly in the knee and hip).

Osteoarthritis (OA): OA is not a single disease but rather the end result of a variety of disorders leading to the structural or functional failure of one or more of your joints. Osteoarthritis involves the entire joint including the nearby muscles, underlying bone, ligaments, joint lining (synovium), and the joint cover (capsule).

Osteotomy: osteotomy ('bone cutting') is a procedure in which a surgeon removes a wedge of bone near a damaged joint. This shifts weight from an area which is damaged to an area where there is a healthier joint surface.

Oxidant: a substance that oxidizes another substance.

Oxidative damage: in the natural process of oxidation (turning oxygen into needed energy), our bodies produce toxins called 'free radicals'. These molecules can cause damage to cells and DNA, but are generally 'mopped up' by substances called antioxidants before they can hurt us.

Pathological: relating to or caused by disease.

Perioperative: relating to, occurring in, or being the period around the time of a surgical operation.

Polyunsaturates: an unsaturated fat is a fat or fatty acid in which there are one or more double bonds in the fatty acid chain. A fat molecule is monounsaturated if it contains one double bond, and polyunsaturated if it contains more than one double bond.

Proximal: nearer to a point of reference such as an origin, a point of attachment, or the midline of the body.

Reflexology: a system of massaging specific areas of the foot or sometimes the hand in order to promote healing, relieve stress, etc. in other parts of the body.

Sclerosis: a thickening or hardening of a body part, such as bone in the joint of someone with OA, especially from excessive formation of fibrous interstitial tissue.

Sciatica: pain along the sciatic nerve usually caused by a herniated disk of the lumbar region of the spine and radiating to the buttocks and to the back of the thigh.

Septic arthritis: infective arthritis may represent a direct invasion of joint space by various microorganisms, including bacteria, viruses, mycobacteria, and fungi.

Synovial joint: a joint so articulated as to move freely.

Synovial capsule: a closed sac of synovial membrane situated between the articular surfaces of joints.

Synovial fluid: a clear fluid secreted by membranes in joint cavities, tendon sheaths, and bursae, and functioning as a lubricant.

Synovium: a thin membrane in synovial (freely moving) joints that lines the joint capsule and secretes synovial fluid.

T'ai chi: an ancient Chinese martial art form that was developed to enhance both physical and emotional well-being.

Tendons: a tendon is a tough yet flexible band of fibrous tissue. the tendon is the structure in your body that connects the muscle to the bones.

Trancutaneous nerve stimulation: transcutaneous electrical nerve stimulation (TENS) involves the passage of low-voltage electrical current to electrodes pasted on the skin.

Valgus: abnormal angulation of a bone or joint, with the angle pointing towards the midline.

Varus: abnormal angulation of a bone or joint, with the angle pointing away from the midline.

Yoga: a system of exercises to promote control of the body and mind.

Index